The Thoracic Surgeon and Emphysema

The Thoracic Surgeon and Emphysema

From Avoidance to Opportunity

David A. Waller

Retired Consultant Thoracic Surgeon
Formerly of Glenfield Hospital
Leicester and St Bartholomew's Hospital
London, UK

WILEY

This edition first published 2027

Registered Offices
John Wiley & Sons, Inc., 111 River Street, Hoboken, NJ 07030, USA
John Wiley & Sons Ltd. New Era House, 8 Oldlands Way, Bognor Regis, West Sussex, PO22 0NO, UK

For details of our global editorial offices, customer services, and more information about Wiley products visit us at www.wiley.com.

The manufacturer's authorized representative according to the EU General Product Safety Regulation is Wiley-VCH GmbH, Boschstr. 12, 69469 Weinheim, Germany, e-mail: Product_Safety@wiley.com.

Wiley also publishes its books in a variety of electronic formats and by print-on-demand. Some content that appears in standard print versions of this book may not be available in other formats.

Library of Congress Cataloging-in-Publication Data has been applied for:

Print ISBN: 9781394380596
ePDF ISBN: 9781394380619
ePUB ISBN: 9781394380602
oBook ISBN: 9781394380626

Cover Design: Wiley
Cover Images: David Waller

Set in 9.5/12.5pt STIXTwoText by Lumina Datamatics

Printed in Singapore
M137330150726

Table of Contents

Preface

Unfortunately, the patient population with tobacco-related lung disease forms the majority of thoracic surgical practice. Whilst lung cancer remains the most common surgical indication, emphysema is the most common comorbidity. The two conditions are inextricably linked by the same aetiology.

Thus, the poor thoracic surgeon has been faced with the threat of emphysema and the risk of its postoperative complications. It is the heart sink which brings the problems of persistent postoperative air leak, prolonged drainage, and hospital stay with increased risk of infective complications and perioperative mortality. Understandably, *avoidance* may be the reason that many patients have been prevented from undergoing thoracic operations, including those for lung cancer, spontaneous pneumothorax, and bullous disease.

The initial pioneers in thoracic surgery for emphysema met with scepticism and scorn. In an era before intensive perioperative care, their endeavours met premature cessation due to poor survival. The reinvention of lung volume reduction surgery (LVRS) some 30 years ago, renovated the revolutionary idea that resection of emphysematous lung tissue could actually improve function. But despite this promise of a remedy to the problems, many were still discouraged by the perceived risk of morbidity and mortality.

The further development of bronchoscopic lung volume reduction around 10 years later inspired a multidisciplinary approach and an increased interest in the medical community, motivated by a less invasive alternative. This had the beneficial, indirect effect of increasing referrals and increasing the use of LVRS.

Surgeons now had a chance to remodel and refresh the damaged lung. There was now an alternative for those who may not have had a disease severe enough or may have been too old to be considered for transplantation. Emphysema could now be viewed as a challenge, not a threat, offering the potential to increase surgical applications extending beyond primarily treating the emphysema. Conventional boundaries of operability for lung cancer surgery could now be challenged. Could emphysema offer a new *opportunity* to the thoracic surgeon?

There did need to be a change in mindset for the Thoracic Surgeon. Surgeons had previously been more concerned with anatomical and pathological elements of thoracic disease. Emphysema surgery required an appreciation of the physiological selection criteria and consequences. The new style thoracic surgeon had much to learn from the respiratory physicians and vice versa. A multidisciplinary approach with important input from radiologists, nuclear medicine specialists, and allied health-care professionals became the template to treat emphysema.

The following chapters will deal with all of the above issues and more. They will be presented in the way that most clinical information is assimilated, by word of mouth. In a series of imaginary dialogues between proponents of LVR and trainees, fellow clinicians in respiratory and transplant medicine, and health-care managers, the main questions surrounding all aspects of LVR will be addressed. Key points will be referenced and illustrated with clinical cases.

The thoracic surgeon who embraces this applied physiology can find it professionally rewarding to find some of the most grateful patients in those who have undergone volume reduction and seen a dramatic improvement in their quality of life. An understanding of the disease can end avoidance and offer new surgical opportunities. Emphysema is your new friend rather than the old foe.

Acknowledgements

I would like to acknowledge the following clinicians who have inspired and helped me in my adventures in lung volume reduction over the last four decades:

Dr Joel Cooper, Thoracic Surgeon, Washington University Hospital, St Louis, who inspired my interest in lung volume reduction surgery for emphysema when I was a young thoracic surgical trainee in the 1990s, with his remarkable presentations.

The Late Mike Morgan, Professor of Respiratory Medicine, Glenfield Hospital, Leicester, who examined me in my final specialist examination and subsequently recruited me as his surgical colleague to develop a lung volume reduction program. I learned so much about respiratory physiology from him, and we applied our knowledge to the benefit of many grateful patients.

The Late Kevin West, Consultant in Cardiothoracic Anaesthesia, Glenfield Hospital, Leicester, whose technical skills and unflappable nature enabled me to operate on patients with emphysema whom every other anaesthetist at the time would have turned down.

The Late Hugoe Matthews, Professor of Thoracic Surgery, Birmingham Heartlands Hospital, who mentored me in my final years of thoracic surgical training and impressed on me the importance of surgical thinking, appreciation of applied physiology, and obtaining all the information in preparation for surgery.

Dr Inger Oey, Clinical Assistant in Thoracic Surgery, Glenfield Hospital, Leicester, whose meticulous data collection and patient follow-up helped to advance our knowledge of lung volume reduction.

My many thoracic surgical trainees whose questions and answers form the basis of many of the imaginary dialogues in this book.

1

Defining the Disease: The "Why"

1.1 Breathlessness

Tutor: "Take a deep breath in and hold it."

Student: "Ugh!"

Now take another breath.

I caaaaan't! (student visibly struggling for breath)

So that's how it feels for a patient with emphysema.

Now, take this heavy book in your hand and stretch out your arm. See how long you can hold it.

After two minutes, the student has to put the book down.

Now try with your elbow bent.

Oh, now that's a lot easier.

Of course, it is because your biceps muscle is working at more mechanical advantage.

Now you understand the physiology of emphysema.

I do?

So, the principle is that the hyperinflated lungs stretch the respiratory muscles such that they respond poorly to the effort of breathing. It is this unrewarded effort that gives the sensation of breathlessness.

But why are the lungs overexpanded or hyperinflated?

Imagine a party balloon and a paper bag.

OK

Your young lungs are like a party balloon, elastic. They empty with little effort. But the emphysematous lung is like a paper bag. The elastic property is lost due to the internal destruction of the alveolar walls.

And is that all down to smoking?

Simplistically, emphysema arises from an induced imbalance between proteases (e.g. neutrophil elastase, MMP-12 and cathepsins) and antiproteases, leading to elastin fibre breakdown. Cigarette smoke or inflammatory cell-derived oxidants or genetic abnormalities (e.g. alpha-1 antitrypsin deficiency) inactivate protease physiologic inhibitors and/or oxidize elastin directly [1].

So, the lung tissue starts to destroy itself?

Yes, and this is an irreversible process leading to airspace enlargement and impaired gas exchange. But also, the loss of elasticity results in mechanical changes, including loss of recoil and airway tension.

So, they struggle to empty their damaged lungs.

Exactly, and when they strain to do so, their airways collapse.

Obstructive airways disease?

Exactly, the classic "church and steeple" flow-volume loop (Figure 1.1). Normal flow, then airways collapse and a reduction in the forced expiratory volume in one second (FEV_1).

A sudden reduction in expiratory flow rate after the initial peak.

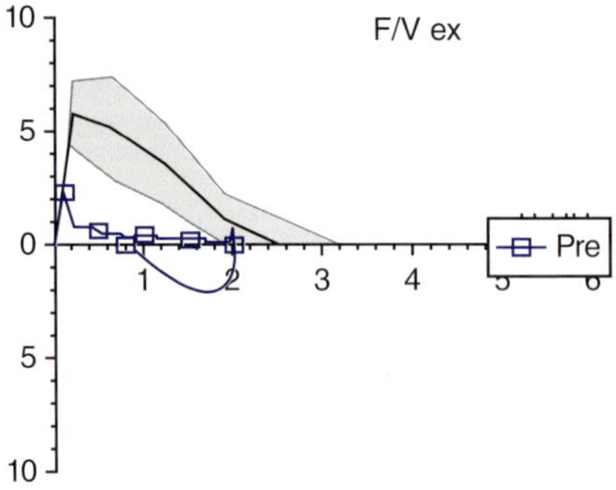

Figure 1.1 The classic flow: volume loop of COPD.

Even worse, because the paper bag is more compliant than the party balloon, it will preferentially fill and continue to trap air as expiration becomes more difficult.

Why is it that patients' activity is limited by breathlessness?

When they experience an increased respiratory rate, such as in exercise or anxiety states, inspiratory tidal volume increases, and expiratory time diminishes further as breathing frequency increases above the baseline value.

So, with every breath, the lung becomes more and more hyperinflated.

Yes, there is a temporary increase in end-expiratory lung volume relative to the resting baseline value. This is "dynamic hyperinflation." The detrimental effects include the following. There is increasing evidence that acute dynamic hyperinflation, when there is worsening expiratory flow-limitation or increased ventilatory demand, can seriously stress cardiopulmonary reserves and increase right ventricular strain [2]. Furthermore, acute-on-chronic dynamic hyperinflation during exercise and COPD exacerbation leads to excessive loading and functional weakness of the inspiratory muscles, which can impose a critical mechanical limitation to ventilation [3].

So, when the emphysema patient exercises, their cardiac function worsens and their respiratory muscles function less well.

Yes, their symptoms can be explained this way.

I have noticed that the emphysema patients try to breathe through pursed lips after they have been walking. Why do they do that?

After minimal exercise, as a result of dynamic hyperinflation, the patient has to rest and try to deflate. The pursed lips act like "auto PEEP" giving some airways positive end-expiratory pressure to attempt to keep the collapsing airways open.

Now I get it!

1.2 Bullae

Let's now think about bullous disease. You are familiar with the situation where an emphysematous bulla may slowly enlarge, occupying more and more of the hemithorax, causing increasing breathlessness?

Yes, absolutely, and in some ways, this has been a more traditional indication for surgery than the more diffuse emphysema treated by lung volume reduction (LVR).

So, how do you explain how the enlarging bulla develops?

Well, it starts with an area of relative weakness in the emphysematous lung, which is fed by a bronchiole and preferentially inflates on inspiration or coughing. Then the small feeding airway acts like a one-way valve as it restricts air outflow.

And how does this bulla lead to breathlessness?

Oh, that's easy. The enlarging bulla compresses and collapses the surrounding lung. This is sometimes described as "vanishing lung syndrome" [4, 5].

So, as you describe "compression," would you think that the pressure inside the bulla is increased relative to its surroundings?

Of course, the air is under tension, which is how it increases in size and compresses the adjacent lung tissue.

Well, I have a surprise for you then. If one measured the pressure inside the bulla, would it be greater, lower or the same as intrapleural pressure?

Obviously greater.

Like a tension pneumothorax?

Oh, perhaps not then.

Because the pressure inside bullae has been measured intraoperatively and...

And?

It has been shown to be negative and similar to pleural pressure [6].

So, if the surrounding lung is not "compressed," then why does it not inflate with inspiration?

The answer is in the relative composition of the alveolar walls of the bulla and the more normal lung. The emphysematous bulla has lost elasticity and, as we stated before, is more like a paper bag than a party balloon and thus fills preferentially. The more elastic surrounding tissue actually retracts and "shrinks away" from the bulla. More of a "pull" than a "push" if you will. There is no real valve-like mechanism, as the bulla has been shown to have a wide airway. However, the loss of elastic recoil may lead to airway collapse on expiration and slower deflation of the bulla.

Why does the bulla lead to breathlessness then?

Possibly due to the extra effort needed in chest wall mechanics to inflate the partially collapsed normal lung. Inflation of the bulla leads to hyperinflation and "overstretching" of the respiratory muscles.

1.3 Phenotypes

Are patients with emphysema a specific group of COPD patients?

Well, it can be a feature of a specific phenotype of COPD.

What is a phenotype?

In this context, a phenotype describes a collection of clinical characteristics such as symptoms, exacerbation frequency, lung function changes or imaging patterns that can be readily identified in clinical practice. Patients can be phenotyped based on changes at the tissue level. One such phenotype is emphysema, which is due to lung tissue destruction [7]. Subgrouping patients into phenotypes emphasizes the fact that COPD is not a single disease but a spectrum of diseases with smoking as a common risk factor [8]. In surgical practice, I like to simplify things and think of three main phenotypes. Can you suggest them?

I am aware of the "pink puffer" and the "blue bloater" descriptions from my old medical school texts.

They still have some relevance, though.

***The emphysematous phenotype* (historically called the "pink puffer," type A) predominantly affects the more elderly, underweight individuals, presenting with pronounced symptoms of dyspnoea but milder inflammation (less cough or sputum production), no cyanosis and arterial blood gas analyses showing a slight decrease in PaO_2 and normal or reduced $PaCO_2$ levels. These patients exhibit extensive alveolar destruction on computed tomography (CT) scans, leading to diminished diffusion capacity and, importantly, pulmonary hyperinflation.**

And the "blue bloater?"

***The chronic bronchitis phenotype* (formerly known as the "blue bloater," type B) is more common in younger, obese individuals and is characterized by pronounced symptoms and inflammation, yet less severe emphysema. It features significant airway obstruction, cyanosis, markedly reduced PaO_2,**

and elevated $PaCO_2$ levels, frequently associated with respiratory failure. Studies indicate that patients with this phenotype of COPD experience more exacerbations.

You said you think of three main phenotypes, what is the third?

***Asthma-COPD overlap (ACO)* also constitutes a clinically significant phenotype, characterized by patients exhibiting features of COPD alongside a history of asthma or evidence of allergy, positive bronchodilator response or eosinophilic inflammation. They may have relatively preserved diffusion capacity but elevated levels of IgE or blood eosinophils. They typically present with persistent airflow obstruction that demonstrates, unlike true COPD, reversible elements (analogous to asthma), with therapeutic implications.**

You mean that patients with this eosinophilic ACO phenotype may respond favourably to inhaled corticosteroid therapy, whereas those with pure emphysema lacking eosinophilic inflammation may not.

Exactly. Furthermore, the more recent therapeutic advances with monoclonal antibodies targeting interleukin 5 (IL-5) or its receptor (IL-5R) have shown benefit in treating this phenotype of COPD [9].

Is a COPD patient only allowed to be one of these phenotypes and not any of the others?

No. An extremely important point. These phenotypes are not mutually exclusive. An individual may be emphysema-dominant but have frequent exacerbations and have features of ACO.

Presumably, this understanding must be taken into consideration when planning therapy, particularly LVR.

Very important. For example, when assessing a patient with a reduced forced expiratory volume and emphysema. The destruction and loss of elastic recoil will reduce the driving pressure through the airway, and the airway may collapse due to a lack of support. However, the resistance to flow may also be affected by small airways inflammation (with mucus plugging) and increased smooth muscle tone.

1.4 COPD as a Healthcare Problem

How common is COPD, do you think?

Well, as we are still seeing the damage of tobacco smoking, there must be millions of cases around the world.

The global prevalence of COPD is thought to be around 10%, and the number affected may reach 600 million by 2050. It is the third highest cause of global mortality, after ischaemic heart disease and cerebrovascular disease [10].

What about in the United Kingdom?

In England, there are around 1.1 million people with a diagnosis of COPD. Around 4.5% of adults over the age of 40 years are living with a diagnosis of COPD, and more than 50% of people currently diagnosed are under 65 years of age. Over 15% are only diagnosed when they present to the hospital as an emergency, and there are an estimated 2,200,000 people with COPD who remain undiagnosed, which is equivalent to 13% of the population of England aged 35 and over [11, 12].

And it must be a major cause of mortality?

The United Kingdom has the 12th highest recorded number of deaths from COPD in the world, with over 30,000 deaths per year and an age-standardized mortality rate of 210.7 deaths per million people between 2001 and 2010 [13]. Fifteen percent of those admitted to the hospital with COPD die within three months, and around 25% die within a year of admission.

What kind of impact does COPD have on the healthcare system?

It is the second most common cause of emergency admissions in the United Kingdom, with an increase of 13% between 2008 and 2014, with an estimated cost of over £1.5 billion per year in direct health care costs [14].

1.5 The Role for Thoracic Surgeons

How many of those with emphysema are suitable for LVR?

In a subset of 959 American patients that represented the part of the general population with advanced emphysema in the pulmonary function database at Beth Israel Deaconess Medical Center, Harvard Medical School, Boston, up to 15% appeared to be potential candidates for LVRS. This estimate was based on a suitable clinical profile plus CT scan evidence of 40% or greater involvement of the lungs and predominantly upper lobe distribution of emphysema [15].

What are the estimates for the United Kingdom?

It has been estimated that of 1.1 million patients with COPD in the United Kingdom, assuming that only 10% of these have severe or very severe

disease and that of these 15% meet the criteria for LVRS [15], this would still make approximately 16,000 potentially eligible for LVR [16].

That sounds like an incredible demand.

A more conservative estimate came from analysis of a primary care database in which 8.1% of patients with COPD met the basic eligibility criteria to consider whether LVRS might be appropriate. If the strictest criteria were applied, including severe dyspnoea with limited co-morbidity and having completed pulmonary rehabilitation, only 0.2% of the COPD population remained eligible [16].

But that is still a lot of potential operations.

Quite. That works out at about 2804 out of 1.3 million patients with COPD in the United Kingdom who could benefit from LVR [17].

Let's find out more about LVR then ...

1.6 Conclusions

The key to the disease process of emphysema is destruction with loss of elasticity leading to distension of the thoracic cavity. So, in some ways, emphysema is more of a chest wall rather than a lung disease. Certainly in terms of surgical treatment it can be viewed that way, and the key structure of interest is actually the diaphragm. The restoration of muscular function and chest wall mechanics is the surgical role in improving the patient's wellbeing.

References

1 Bentaher A, Glehen O, Degobert G. Pulmonary emphysema: current understanding of disease pathogenesis and therapeutic approaches. Biomedicines. 2025;13(9):2120.
2 Welling JBA, Slebos DJ. Dynamics of hyperinflation. Respirology. 2023;28(6): 507–508. https://doi.org/10.1111/resp.14507
3 O'Donnell DE, Laveneziana P. The clinical importance of dynamic lung hyperinflation in COPD. COPD. 2006;3(4):219–232.
4 Sharma N, Justaniah AM, Kanne JP, Gurney JW, Mohammed TL. Vanishing lung syndrome (giant bullous emphysema): CT findings in 7 patients and a literature review. J Thorac Imaging. 2009;24(3):227–230.
5 Faruqi S, Varma R. The vanishing lung: an important cause of hyperlucency on chest radiograph. Acute Med. 2013;12(3):159–162.

6 Morgan MD, Edwards CW, Morris J, Matthews HR. Origin and behaviour of emphysematous bullae. Thorax. 1989;44(7):533–538.

7 Xie C, Wang K, Yang K, Zhong Y, Gul A, Luo W, et al. Toward precision medicine in COPD: phenotypes, endotypes, biomarkers, and treatable traits. Respir Res. 2025 Sep 29;26(1):274.

8 Yousuf A, McAuley H, Elneima O, Brightling CE. The different phenotypes of COPD. Br Med Bull. 2021;137(1):82–97.

9 Donovan T, Milan SJ, Wang R, Banchoff E, Bradley P, Crossingham I. Anti-IL-5 therapies for chronic obstructive pulmonary disease. Cochrane Database Syst Rev. 2020;12(12):CD013432.

10 The Global Initiative for Chronic Obstructive Lung Disease (GOLD) report 2025. https://goldcopd.org/2025-gold-report/

11 Nacul L, Soljak M, Samarasundera E, Hopkinson NS, Lacerda E, Indulkar T, et al. COPD in England: a comparison of expected, model-based prevalence and observed prevalence from general practice data. J Pub Health. 2010;(33):108–116.

12 Scholes S, Moody A, Mindell JS. Estimating population prevalence of potential airflow obstruction using different spirometric criteria: a pooled cross-sectional analysis of persons aged 40-95 years in England and Wales. BMJ Open. 2014; 4(7):e005685

13 Chronic obstructive pulmonary disease in over 16s: diagnosis and management. NICE guideline 2019. https://www.nice.org.uk/guidance/ng115

14 McLean S, Hoogendoorn M, Hoogenveen RT et al. Projecting the COPD population and costs in England and Scotland: 2011 to 2030. Sci Rep. 2016;6:31893.

15 Akuthota P. An evidence-based estimate on the size of the potential patient pool for lung volume reduction surgery. Ann Thorac Surg. 2012;94(1):205–211.

16 Clark SJ, Zoumot Z, Bamsey O, Polkey MI, Dusmet M, Lim E, et al. Surgical approaches for lung volume reduction in emphysema. Clin Med (Lond). 2014; 14(2):122–127.

17 Whittaker HR, Connell O, Campbell J, Elbehairy AF, Hopkinson NS, Quint JK. Eligibility for lung volume reduction surgery in patients with COPD identified in a UK primary care setting. Chest. 2020;157(2):276–285. https://doi.org/10.1016/j.chest.2019.07.016

2

Defining the Interventions: The "How"

2.1 History

Trainee: So, how did the concept that resecting lung tissue could possibly improve lung function arise?

Trainer: The principle, first described by Otto Brantigan in the 1950s, was to surgically resect or exclude, by incision and oversewing, the most functionless lung tissue to reduce the volume of the emphysematous lung to that in expiration for the normal lung [1].

So, the procedure did not take off because of the high mortality.

Exactly, and it was not until Joel Cooper resurrected the technique in the 1990s, using mechanical linear staplers to resect, that the operation of lung volume reduction surgery (LVRS) entered practice again [2].

How did he think of looking for this historical report?

I believe it was based on the improvements seen in patients undergoing single-lung transplant for emphysema, even in the face of initial graft dysfunction. The "volume reduction effect" of the smaller transplanted lung gave mechanical benefit before any gas exchange improvement was obtained.

So, was the procedure of LVRS restricted to transplant candidates in the initial phase?

No, not exclusively. Cooper was very meticulous regarding selection and perioperative care. The principles of which have continued to form the basis of modern-day selection (see Chapter 3). But he did advocate bilateral LVRS via median sternotomy as a single procedure.

That sounds like an extensive undertaking for a patient with severely limited lung function.

It was, but at that time, video-assisted thoracoscopic surgery was developing, and it was an obvious application of minimally invasive techniques. Initially, not only stapled lung resection but also peripheral laser ablation was used. However, VATS resection evolved as the approach of choice [3], and there began a debate around whether a one-stage bilateral or a staged unilateral approach was preferable [4]. But we will discuss that controversy, which persists until the present day, later in Chapter 4.

When did endobronchial LVR start to enter clinical practice?

One of the earliest reports of endobronchial occlusion to provoke LVR by lobar collapse originated from Bradford, United Kingdom [5]. Simple silicone bronchial blockers were used to good effect. The initial use of a one-way endobronchial valve appeared in 2003 in London [6]. This Zephyr valve was then taken through several randomized trials to establish its benefits over medical therapy. We will discuss these in more detail in Chapter 5.

Was the use of LVRS tested in a randomized trial?

The initial use of LVRS, of course, predated the advent of EBLVR, and indeed, the reports by Cooper prompted rapid adoption of the technique in the United States. So much so that a temporary moratorium was placed pending further trial evaluation. This was because there was somewhat indiscriminate use of the technique, leading to a flood of claims for reimbursement but a need for clearer selection criteria.

And that was the National Emphysema Treatment Trial (NETT)?

Yes, the NETT was one of the largest randomized thoracic surgical trials ever completed [7]. One thousand two hundred and eighteen patients with severe emphysema were randomized to either bilateral LVRS or continued medical treatment.

LVRS gave a survival advantage for patients with both predominantly upper-lobe emphysema and low baseline exercise capacity, but those with non-upper-lobe emphysema and high baseline exercise had increased mortality and negligible functional gain. But its findings had many implications for selection (more later in Chapter 3).

2.2 Mechanism of LVR

But how can surgery help in these very sick patients? How can resecting lung tissue possibly improve their lung function and not simply leave them to die in respiratory failure on a mechanical ventilator?

Excision or exclusion of the most damaged emphysematous lung tissue removes the most compliant parts of the lung and restores the overall elastic recoil [8]. This is the analogy of "darning a ladder in a nylon stocking."

Perhaps a little dated nowadays...

But you understand that removing the area of weakness and increasing the elastic strength of the lung tissue (the driving pressure) means less air is trapped in the lungs after expiration. It also increases the "pull" on the airways, decreases airway collapse and increases airway conductance [9].

So, they become less hyperinflated.

Yes, their residual volume is reduced and thus the overstretching of the respiratory muscles. Breathing is more efficient, the effort is more rewarded and the sense of breathlessness is diminished. So, an improvement in respiratory mechanics counteracts any loss of gas-exchanging lung tissue. There may also be an improvement in right ventricular function [10].

How does LVR improve cardiac function?

The reduction of hyperinflation using either EBLVR or LVRS significantly improves venous return, cardiac preload, myocardial contractility and cardiac output, without changes in pulmonary artery pressures [11, 12].

And the improvements in cardiorespiratory function lead to an increased exercise tolerance.

It was found that patients adopted a slower, deeper breathing pattern during exercise after LVRS, and understandably, as we explained in Chapter 1, this correlated with a reduction in dynamic hyperinflation [13]. This reduction, in turn, was associated with an increased 6-minute walk distance. As expected, improved respiratory muscle strength due to the reduction in hyperinflation also correlated with improved exercise performance [14].

But why does the patient with a successful LVR outcome feel less breathless?

Firstly, it causes an increased elastic recoil, which at least partially explains the enhanced maximal expiratory flow. Secondly, it is associated with a reduction of hyperinflation, which allows for an increase in global inspiratory muscle strength and in diaphragmatic contribution to tidal volume as well as a decrease in the inspiratory elastic load imposed by the chest wall. Taken together, these effects result in a reduced work of breathing and in an enhanced maximal ventilation, which both contribute to the increased exercise capacity and reduced dyspnoea after surgery [15].

What affects the work of breathing (WOB)?

Dynamic hyperinflation increases the WOB on inspiration due to impaired inspiratory muscle function, particularly the diaphragm. These muscles are forced to work at an unfavourable length for pressure generation due to the overstretching of hyperinflation. Put simply, more effort is required to get the same result. A persistently increased WOB results in respiratory muscle fatigue [16].

So, the diaphragm is all-important in LVR.

Yes, I think improving the contour of the diaphragm is the main objective of LVR in emphysema. So, in patient selection, the key aim is to start with a flattened diaphragmatic contour on the chest X-ray, which regains its normal curve contour postoperatively. This radiographic image represents an increase in transdiaphragmatic pressure, which is lost in a hyperinflated lung and whose improvement correlates with improved exercise capacity [14].

But what the patient is looking for is an actual improvement in quality of life.

Exercise limitation is one of the main causes of impaired quality of life in these patients suffering from severe emphysema [17]. But this specific improvement can lead to multifactorial improvements in lifestyle for many years after both LVRS and EBLVR.

How long can these benefits last?

There are reports that at 12 months after LVRS, physical functioning, role limitations due to physical health and vitality reached statistical significance [18]. Furthermore, we found that in an intentional staged programme of sequential unilateral LVR procedures, using a combination of LVRS and EBLVR, there was a sustained improvement over baseline in the health status measures: EuroQol-5D, which improved from 50 ± 26 to 62 ± 23 ($P < 0.01$) for up to 5 years and the Short Form 36-item

(SF 36) questionnaire for up to 9 years. Specifically, within the SF 36 results, role limitations because of physical health problems were significantly improved for up to 7 years, with similar benefits in social functioning and energy levels for 8 and 9 years, respectively [19].

2.3 What Are the Best Ways to Measure the Benefits of LVR?

Having heard the various benefits of LVR, why is it that the success of the treatment seems to be judged by improvements in spirometry?

The most commonly used outcome measure (possibly because it is the easiest to measure) has been improvement in the obstructive element of emphysema, the change in forced expiratory volume in one second (FEV_1), which should improve if airway collapse is reduced by removing the least elastic parts of the lung. However, only about 15% of patients in the only randomized controlled trial (CELEB) [20] achieved the minimal clinically important difference (MCID) in FEV_1 after either LVRS or EBLVR.

Oh, that's quite disappointing at only 15%.

Not really, when you consider that patients with emphysema will seldom come into your clinic and say, "Doctor, my FEV_1 feels a bit lower today."

OK, I get what you mean.

The assumption that only by improving FEV_1 can one improve the course of the disease may not be relevant in LVR. The use of a multidimensional measure is considered a more meaningful way to evaluate prognosis and response to disease-modifying interventions than FEV_1 alone [21].

Which measure is best, do you think?

The B-O-D-E index that creates a score between 0 (the best health) and 10 (the worst) is calculated on four commonly used COPD outcome measures: BMI, FEV_1, modified MRC score, and 6-minute walk distance. Sometimes, the incremental shuttle walk distance is used to generate the iBODE score. It includes *objective* measures of the disease impact on lung function, the "O" (FEV_1% predicted) and 6-minute walk distance, the "E" (6MWT), a *subjective* patient-reported outcome reflecting the patients' perception of dyspnoea (mMRC score), the "D" and the body mass index, the "B" which reflects the *systemic* involvement of COPD.

Why do you prefer this index?

As we have discussed in Chapter 1, COPD is a heterogeneous collection of several clinical phenotypes that can overlap; therefore, the combination of several indices in the BODE index should have better prognostic value than any isolated variable specific to only one phenotype [22].

And by how much does LVR improve the BODE index?

After one-stage bilateral LVRS, the BODE index in higher-risk patients showed a decrease from 7.2 +/− 1.6 preoperatively to 4.0 +/− 2.0 at 3 months [23]. In lower-risk patients undergoing unilateral LVRS, the BODE index improved from a median of 5 (interquartile range 4–5) before surgery to 3 (interquartile range 2–4) 1 year after surgery. A lower preoperative 6-minute walk distance predicted a greater improvement in the BODE index after 1 year [24]. After EBLVR, the BODE index showed a significant lasting improvement with 86% improved at one year and 71% at 2 years follow-up [25].

Having said all of this, I still feel that we should measure the outcome of LVR by how much it has changed the patient's life. Therefore, although they are time-consuming to collect, I think that detailed health status questionnaires are the best assessment. The motivation of the patient is something that cannot be objectively assessed but which undoubtedly affects the outcome of LVR. I tell them that reducing hyperinflation will improve their capacity to do more, but unless you push yourself to new limits, you will not feel the full benefit.

2.4 How Frequently Is LVR Used to Treat Severe Emphysema?

The answer is: nowhere near as often as it should be.

Why isn't LVR more commonly used?

I think that this is where the "Fear Factor" comes into play. In the United States, in the opinion of leading pulmonologists, "lung volume reduction surgery has largely fallen out of favour given high perioperative risk, complex patient selection and few centres offering the procedure" [26]. Although more hope is portrayed for EBLVR. However, it is reported that since 2011, national LVRS utilization has been increasing with decreasing mortality rates. At the hospital level, six hospitals performed 40% of all

LVRS nationally, with an adjusted national 30-day mortality rate of 4.3% and composite outcome rate of 15.8%.

What only six centres in the entire United States?

Yes, the remaining 40% of LVRS was performed amongst 159 lower-volume centres.

What are the reasons for this apparent postcode lottery?

This inequity of access may be attributed to the eligibility criteria for reimbursement. Apparently, the Center for Medicare and Medicaid Services (CMS) lists three types of facilities that are eligible for reimbursement for LVRS: (1) NETT trial participants; (2) centres credentialed by the Joint Commission on Accreditation of Healthcare Organizations under their Disease Specific Certification Program for LVRS; and (3) Medicare approved for lung or heart and lung transplants. Which is obviously an exclusive club. The adjusted outcomes were found to be similar across all hospitals, which hopefully will stimulate revision of this rationing policy [27].

You mentioned the "Fear Factor."

Unfortunately, the older results from the initial NETT study may have changed referral practices for LVRS. Pulmonologists and other referring providers may have been dissuaded by their perception of risk. In the United Kingdom, a survey by the British Thoracic Society of their members revealed that estimates for a post-LVRS 30-day mortality were 0–5% in 52% of respondents, 21% overestimated this and 27% did not know. A third of the respondents thought that more than 10% of patients would be in hospital 1-month post procedure, and 28% were unsure [28].

How were these attitudes reflected in UK practice?

Hospital activity analysis showed that in the 5-year period 2017–2022, there were just over 1500 LVR procedures performed in England (NHS England, personal communication). These were concentrated in two or three main regions, with something of a "postcode lottery" in effect, where the geographic origin of the patient determined their likelihood of receiving LVR treatment.

What was the official response to these figures?

To address any doubts of the healthcare providers, NHS England agreed to the routine commissioning of both LVRS and EBLVR with the Zephyr valve across all regions (NHS Clinical Commissioning Policy 1622).

And only time will tell if these reassurances allayed the innate “Fear of LVR” in the referrers.

Hopefully, as we shall see in the following chapters, this fear is misplaced and careful selection and individualized risk assessment can give the thousands of eligible patients with emphysema access to LVR services.

2.5 Conclusions

The concept of lung volume reduction to treat emphysema is nearly 70 years old. It developed as an extension of the operation of bullectomy with removal of more surrounding damaged lung tissue. However, it was not until the modern era with improved perioperative care and the scientific rigour of the randomized trial that its place became established.

I believe that the prime mechanism of benefit is in improved respiratory mechanics, especially in restoring diaphragmatic function. Improvements in pulmonary haemodynamics are likely to be secondary to redistribution of ventilation, capillary recruitment and reduction in vascular resistance.

The technology of bronchoscopic approaches was developed to allay fears of the risk of surgery, yet their advent may have increased referrals for both methods.

References

1 Brantigan OC, Mueller E. Surgical treatment of pulmonary emphysema. Am Surg. 1957;23(9):789–804.
2 Cooper JD, Trulock EP, Triantafillou AN, Patterson GA, Pohl MS, Deloney PA, et al. Bilateral pneumectomy (volume reduction) for chronic obstructive pulmonary disease. J Thorac Cardiovasc Surg. 1995;109(1):106–116.
3 McKenna RJ Jr, Brenner M, Gelb AF, Mullin M, Singh N, Peters H, et al. A randomized, prospective trial of stapled lung reduction versus laser bullectomy for diffuse emphysema. J Thorac Cardiovasc Surg. 1996;111(2):317–321; discussion 322.
4 McKenna RJ Jr, Brenner M, Fischel RJ, Gelb AF. Should lung volume reduction for emphysema be unilateral or bilateral? J Thorac Cardiovasc Surg. 1996;112(5):1331–1338; discussion 1338–1339.
5 Sabanathan S, Richardson J, Pieri-Davies S. Bronchoscopic lung volume reduction. J Cardiovasc Surg (Torino). 2003;44(1):101–108.
6 Toma TP, Hopkinson NS, Hillier J, Hansell DM, Morgan C, Goldstraw PG, et al. Bronchoscopic volume reduction with valve implants in patients with severe emphysema. Lancet. 2003;361(9361):931–933.

7 Fishman A, Martinez F, Naunheim K, Piantadosi S, Wise R, Ries A, et al. A randomized trial comparing lung-volume-reduction surgery with medical therapy for severe emphysema. N Engl J Med. 2003;348(21):2059–2073.

8 Gelb AF, McKenna RJ Jr, Brenner M, Fischel R, Baydur A, Zamel N. Contribution of lung and chest wall mechanics following emphysema resection. Chest. 1996;110(1):11–17.

9 Gelb AF, Zamel N, McKenna RJ Jr, Brenner M. Mechanism of short-term improvement in lung function after emphysema resection. Am J Respir Crit Care Med. 1996; 154(4 Pt 1):945–951. https://doi.org/10.1164/ajrccm.154.4.8887590

10 Sciurba FC, Rogers RM, Keenan RJ, Slivka WA, Gorcsan J 3rd, Ferson PF, et al. Improvement in pulmonary function and elastic recoil after lung-reduction surgery for diffuse emphysema. N Engl J Med. 1996;334:1095–1099.

11 van der Molen MC, Hartman JE, Vanfleteren LEGW, Kerstjens HAM, van Melle JP, Willems TP, et al. Reduction of lung hyperinflation improves cardiac preload, contractility, and output in emphysema: a clinical trial in patients who received endobronchial valves. Am J Respir Crit Care Med. 2022;206(6):704–711.

12 Criner GJ, Scharf SM, Falk JA, Gaughan JP, Sternberg AL, Patel NB, et al. Effect of lung volume reduction surgery on resting pulmonary hemodynamics in severe emphysema. Am J Respir Crit Care Med. 2007;176(3):253–260.

13 Lammi, MR, Marchetti, N, Criner, GJ. Reduced dynamic hyperinflation after LVRS is associated with improved exercise tolerance. Respir Med. 2014 108(10): 1491–1497.

14 Criner G, Cordova FC, Leyenson V, Roy B, Travaline J, Sudarshan S, et al. Effect of lung volume reduction surgery on diaphragm strength. Am J Respir Crit Care Med. 1998;157(5 Pt 1):1578–1585.

15 Marchand E, Gayan-Ramirez G, De Leyn P, Decramer M. Physiological basis of improvement after lung volume reduction surgery for severe emphysema: where are we? Eur Respir J. 1999;13(3):686–696.

16 Tschernko EM, Gruber EM, Jaksch P, Jandrasits O, Jantsch U, Brack T, et al. Ventilatory mechanics and gas exchange during exercise before and after lung volume reduction surgery. Am J Respir Crit Care Med. 1998; 158(5 Pt 1): 1424–1431.

17 Gallagher CG. Exercise and chronic obstructive pulmonary disease. Med Clin North Am. 1990;74(3):619–641.

18 Seadler B, Thuppal S, Rizvi N, Markwell S, Sawyer J, McCullough K, et al. Clinical and quality of life outcomes after lung volume reduction surgery. Ann Thorac Surg. 2019;108(3):866–872.

19 Oey I, Steiner M, Morgan M, Waller D. Patient-directed volume reduction for emphysema: Sequential surgical and endobronchial techniques. Ann Thorac Surg. 2021;112(1):295–301.

20 Buttery SC, Banya W, Bilancia R, Boyd E, Buckley J, Greening NJ, et al. Lung volume reduction surgery versus endobronchial valves: a randomised controlled trial. Eur Respir J. 2023;61(4):2202063.

21 Celli BR. Change in the BODE index reflects disease modification in COPD: lessons from lung volume reduction surgery. Chest. 2006;129(4):835–836.

22 Corlateanu A, Plahotniuc A, Corlateanu O, Botnaru V, Bikov A, Mathioudakis AG, et al. Multidimensional indices in the assessment of chronic obstructive pulmonary disease. Respir Med. 2021; 185:106519.

23 Imfeld S, Bloch KE, Weder W, Russi EW. The BODE index after lung volume reduction surgery correlates with survival. Chest. 2006;129(4):873–878.

24 Lederer DJ, Thomashow BM, Ginsburg ME, Austin JH, Bartels MN, Yip CK, et al. Lung-volume reduction surgery for pulmonary emphysema: improvement in body mass index, airflow obstruction, dyspnoea, and exercise capacity index after 1 year. J Thorac Cardiovasc Surg. 2007;133(6):1434–1438.

25 Bivort D, Blondeel A, Geysen H, Vandervelde CM, Coolen J, Ceulemans LJ, et al. Two-year results of bronchoscopic lung volume reduction using one-way endobronchial valves: real-world single center data. Int J Chron Obstruct Pulmon Dis. 2025;20:799–810.

26 Kapp CM, Kalhan R. The quest for safe and effective bronchoscopic lung volume reduction – a matter of correct scaffolding? Am J Respir Crit Care Med. 2025;211(7):1110–1112.

27 Abdelsattar ZM, Allen M, Blackmon S, Cassivi S, Mandrekar J, Nichols F, et al. Contemporary practice patterns of lung volume reduction surgery in the United States. Ann Thorac Surg. 2021;112(3):952–960.

28 McNulty W, Jordan S, Hopkinson NS. Attitudes and access to lung volume reduction surgery for COPD – a survey by the British Thoracic Society. BMJ Open Respiratory Research. 2014;1:e000023.

3

Case Selection: Do You Feel Lucky?

Trainee: But surely not all patients with emphysema are suitable for lung volume reduction (LVR)?

Trainer: Well, selection of those who will benefit most with acceptable risk is the most challenging but rewarding aspect of this surgery. The risks can be high, but the treatment can be potentially life-changing for the patient.

Are there any basic principles in selection for LVR?

Yes, I like to think of "The 3 Bs"

Well Breathless...and Big Lungs?

Excellent. And *Bad enough* to want something doing about it.

3.1 Physiology

Ok, so big lungs mean they are hyperinflated with a large residual volume (RV).

Yes, the more hyperinflated, the better but in our experience anRV > 180% of predicted with a ratio to total lung capacity (RV:TLC) of over 57%. It is important to note that these static lung volumes: RV and TLC should be measured using body box plethysmography rather than relying on helium dilution methods. The latter requires adequate ventilation of all parts of the lung, which is not the case in severe emphysema and may therefore lead to an underestimation of lung volumes.

Is there a strict cut-off for "significant" hyperinflation?

As we discussed in Chapter 1, many of the patients' symptoms of exercise limitation may be related to dynamic hyperinflation, worsening the

existing static hyperinflation. So, it has been suggested [1] that those with static hyperinflation lower than the currently accepted treatment selection threshold of RV 175% of predicted or RV/TLC ratio of >55% could be clinical responders after LVR.

Breathlessness must be due to chronic obstructive pulmonary disease (COPD), so their forced expiratory volume in one second (FEV_1) must be reduced?

Of course, but there is always variability in this measurement, so it is difficult to be didactic. A value below 20% predicted is indicative of severe disease, and the risk needs to be taken into account. On the other hand, a value of FEV_1 above 50% predicted may suggest another cause for the breathlessness. However, as we shall see, none of these parameters can be taken in isolation. This is because, as we discussed in Chapter 1, COPD is a heterogeneous collection of different phenotypes that may overlap.

What other physiological parameters are important in selection for LVR?

Well, markers of the severity of the emphysema in the patient are paramount. Loss of diffusion capacity (DLCO) may increase the risk of any intervention and reduce the response. Levels below 20% of predicted are indicators of risk.

Presumably, gas exchange suffers if diffusion capacity falls.

Yes, so signs of type II respiratory failure are relative contraindications to LVR. Chronic levels of arterial pCO_2 above 55 mmHg or 7.5 kPa, despite nocturnal ventilation, suggest that the patient may struggle to tolerate the procedure and recover from the anaesthetic or may need mechanical ventilation afterwards.

What about type I respiratory failure and patients with hypoxia?

Yes, this is a relative contraindication, particularly as it is associated with pulmonary hypertension. As a "rule of thumb," I would exclude a patient from LVR if their pO_2 was less than their pCO_2. However, some have extended the boundaries of selection into those with hypercapnia who may be using non-invasive ventilation already [2].

How important is a measurement of pulmonary hypertension?

Certainly, echocardiography is mandatory before accepting anyone for LVR. But can you think of any problems in these patients due to their emphysema?

Does the hyperinflation not affect the ultrasound examination?

Indeed, so transthoracic estimation of pulmonary hypertension is likely to be inaccurate due to suboptimal windows through the air trapping. I prefer to look for evidence of right ventricular dysfunction. Can you explain why this would be a worry in those undergoing LVR?

Any resection of lung tissue will reduce the pulmonary vascular bed and increase pulmonary vascular resistance (PVR), thus increasing afterload and strain on the right ventricle.

That is possible, although it has been argued that this effect of an anatomically reduced vascular bed after LVR surgery (LVRS) may be counterbalanced by a decrease in PVR.

How is that possible?

By reducing hyperinflation and increasing elastic recoil, the improved mechanical properties of the lung may cause less functional compression and hence increased capillary recruitment [3].

So, is pulmonary hypertension a relative contraindication to LVR?

Yes, it is a grey area; however, some centres have reported successful LVRS and endobronchial LVR (EBLVR) in those with moderate pulmonary hypertension [4, 5]. I think that with established pulmonary hypertension, together with signs of right ventricular dysfunction, one should consider referral for lung transplantation rather than LVR.

So that is why Brantigan advised targeting the most "functionless" lung (see Chapter 2)?

Yes, so that is why target selection is of prime importance. Reduction in hyperinflation by excluding functionless tissue with preservation of gas-exchanging functioning parenchyma is the basic objective of lung volume reduction.

3.2 Targets

And some of the most damaged emphysematous lung is relatively useless?

Yes, that's right. Emphysema is predominantly a disease of the peripheral lung tissue, creating targets of poorly perfused areas, which can be resected to achieve volume reduction without significantly affecting gas exchange.

So, is the opposite situation called non-heterogeneous or I suppose homogeneous?

Yes, so-called homogeneous emphysema is a common exclusion criterion and a reason to advise against LVR. But I don't think it is as simple as that.

You mean it is not a question of heterogeneous or homogeneous?

No, it is not a simple dichotomy. Emphysema is not a lobar disease (except in severe alpha-1 anti-trypsin deficiency), it is primarily a peripheral lung disease and may well be patchy within a lobe. There may be *intralobar heterogeneity* as well as *interlobar heterogeneity*. This is most obvious on the perfusion scan and particularly on a single-photon emission computed tomography (SPECT) scan, which may enable identification of targets in three dimensions (3D).

What is a SPECT scan?

The standard method of assessment has been planar ventilation/perfusion scintigraphy (Figure 3.5) with technetium-labelled albumin particles (Tc-99m-MAA). SPECT is a nuclear medicine tomographic imaging technique using gamma rays [6]. It is similar to the conventional planar imaging but is able to provide relative lobar perfusion data with superior spatial resolution by allowing 3D perfusion registration and fusion with a low-dose CT for spatial anatomy.

And does this influence the choice of treatment?

Yes, there may be little interlobar heterogeneity, making EBLVR less suitable, as this involves the exclusion of an entire lobe. However, areas of intralobar heterogeneity may be amenable to targeted LVRS if only the peripheries of the lobe are underperfused.

I guess that EBLVR is dependent on "lobar" targets.

Non-response to EBV treatment is associated with a less-than-ideal or non-optimal target lobe, based on emphysema, perfusion and air trapping. These non-responders had significantly less destruction, less air trapping and higher perfusion in the target lobe compared to the responder clusters [7]. We will discuss non-response to EBLVR in more detail in Chapter 7.

Is there a clear definition of when the disease is too homogeneous to consider LVR?

Not really, as there are series reported where significant benefits have been found from both LVRS and EBLVR. However, some suggest that the function, or perfusion, of the target lobe should not exceed 20% of overall perfusion [8].

But what is the best method of target selection?

A thin-slice (1 mm) high-resolution CT scan without contrast enhancement will allow assessment of the severity of emphysema.

And how can you assess the CT images to select for LVR?

A variety of commercially available software tools (Figure 3.1) can be used for lobe-based quantification using an attenuation threshold of –950 HU for measuring emphysema for thin-section CT scans. A threshold of –910 HU is also used by some software, which reports both thresholds and may be more sensitive for detecting less severe emphysema.

How important is this threshold in Hounsfield Units (HU)?

The nearer the value to –1000 HU, the nearer the density of the lung tissue to air, so the more severe the extent of emphysema. Therefore, assessments at –910 HU can include some small airways disease-associated gas trapping in their measurements, as the lung is not severely damaged. However, the majority of the trial evidence for EBLVR comes from using

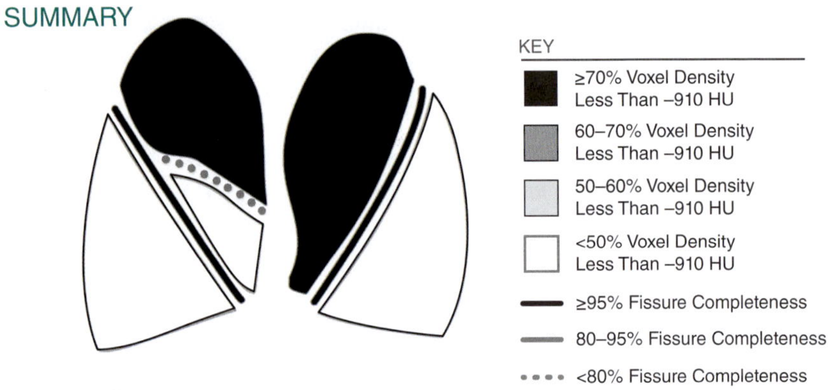

RESULTS

	RIGHT LUNG				LEFT LUNG	
	RUL	RUL + RML	RML	RLL	LUL	LLL
% Fissure Completeness	96.7	–1.0	–1.0	96.7	98.4	98.4
% Voxel Density Less Than –910 HU	77	–1	–1	20	72	17
% Voxel Density Less Than –950 HU	60	–1	–1	11	56	9
Inspiratory Volume (ml)	1699	–1	–1	1009	1449	807

Figure 3.1 StratX® software analysis of CT thorax.

assessments at −910 HU for patient selection. The most common cutoffs for lobe destruction are: at least 30% of the target lobe with −950 HU cutoff or at least 40–50% of the target lobe with −910 HU cutoff in the absence of other significant lung disease (e.g. fibrosis, bronchiectasis) [9].

How do you interpret the targets on the quantitative CT?

Firstly, the lobar voxel density measurements give an idea of the likely lobar targets. But this assessment must be correlated with the estimated lobar volume. A high emphysema severity (measured at −950 or −910 HU) must correlate with the largest lobar volume.

It is important to note that there may be problems in interpreting the quantitative CT scans. Sometimes the destruction score (DS) may seem lower than expected (Figure 3.2). There can be several reasons for this

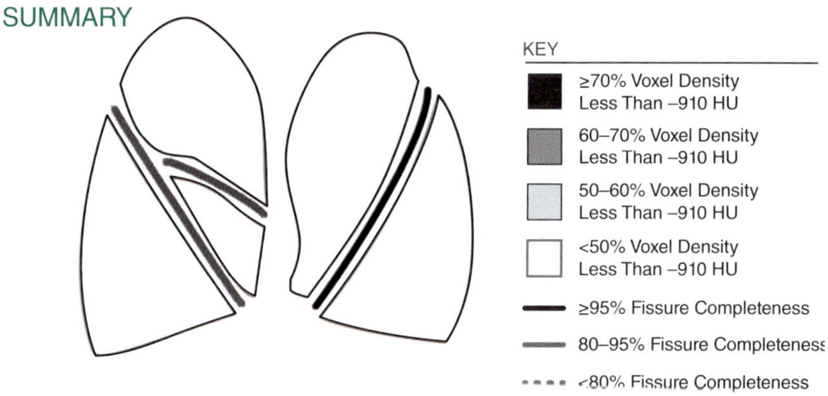

RESULTS

	RIGHT LUNG				LEFT LUNG	
	RUL	RUL + RML	RML	RLL	LUL	LLL
% Fissure Completeness	82.4	89.4	90.0	89.4	100.0	100.0
% Voxel Density Less Than −910 HU	12	15	40	29	10	6
% Voxel Density Less Than −950 HU	1	2	10	5	1	0
Inspiratory Volume (ml)	1903	2126	223	910	1782	1125

Figure 3.2 A StratX® report with lower-than-expected DS in a patient with severe emphysema and clinically suitable for LVR.

anomaly. Air trapping, small airway disease or other conditions can lead to a high RV and low FEV_1 without emphysema destruction. The diseased lobe may contain emphysema but may not quite reach 50% at −910 HU. "Noisy" scans can have artefacts presenting as light-coloured voxels (air should be black) in the air spaces outside of the patient and in the trachea, which may lower the DS. If there appears to be a discrepancy between the clinical picture and the imaging report, then the scan should be repeated.

But does the severity of emphysema equate to loss of function?

In general, the most severely emphysematous lung will be the least perfused, but I would always want to correlate the CT findings with a quantitative lung perfusion scan [6].

Surely, the most severely emphysematous lobes of the lung are most poorly perfused.

We tried to correlate the values obtained for emphysema severity and lobar perfusion using the StratX values for −910 HU and the estimated percentage lobar perfusion on SPECT. There was a clear correlation in the upper five segments on the right and left, but no correlation for either lower lobe (Figures 3.3 and 3.4).

What causes are there for the discrepancy between the emphysema DS and the perfusion measurements?

In Figure 3.5, the least perfused lobe was not emphysematous but was destroyed secondary to pulmonary fibrosis. If this lobe had been targeted

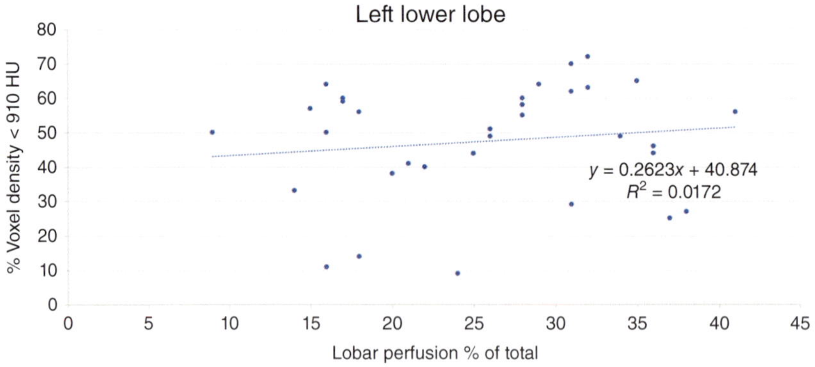

Figure 3.3 The relationship of lobar perfusion and emphysema severity in the left lower lobe.

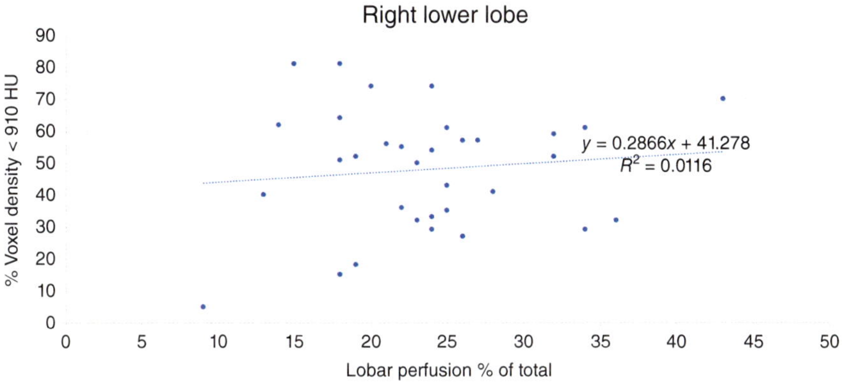

Figure 3.4 The relationship of lobar perfusion and emphysema severity in the right lower lobe.

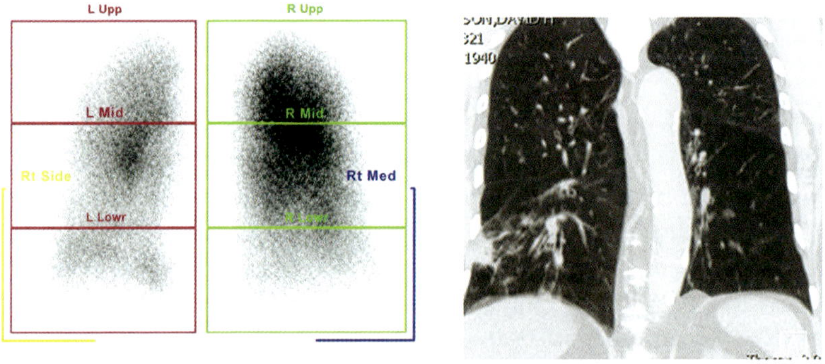

POSTERIOR

(% Ratios)	Left	Right
Upper	12.36	20.54
Middle	18.13	31.37
Lower	8.32	9.28
Total	38.81	61.19

ANTERIOR

(% Ratios)	Left	Right
Upper	15.71	22.31
Middle	19.81	29.26
Lower	5.79	7.11
Total	41.32	58.68

Figure 3.5 Quantitative lung perfusion scan suggests bilateral lower lobe targets, but the CT demonstrates right lower lobe fibrosis and volume loss.

for LVR, then the patient's condition would have worsened. The remaining emphysematous lung would have received increased ventilation, and thus the hyperinflation would have worsened. On the other hand, a lobe may seem well perfused but may still contain a significant area of destroyed tissue, as the value is an average for the whole lobe. There may still be a target for LVRS.

Do you think that this understanding about the need to correlate anatomical and functional imaging has always been applied correctly in the literature?

Unfortunately not. In the National Emphysema Treatment Trial (NETT), there was some inaccuracy in the definition of upper vs lower lobe predominant disease: Among 284 of 1045 patients with low exercise capacity at baseline and upper lobe–predominant emphysema on CT, 202 patients had low upper zone perfusion and lower mortality with LVRS vs medical management (risk ratio [RR], 0.56; $P = 0.008$) [8].

Yes, this was the important finding about which group received a survival benefit from LVRS.

However, the remaining 82 patients (29%) had high perfusion and no mortality benefit (RR, 0.97; $P = 0.62$). Similarly, among 404 of 1045 patients with upper lobe-predominant emphysema and high exercise capacity, 126 (31%) had high perfusion, and there was no benefit from LVRS (RR, 1.05; $P = 1.00$). Overall, of 688 with upper lobe-predominant emphysema on CT, 208 (30.2%) had high (>20%) upper zone perfusion [8]. A post hoc analysis of the NETT recommended that patients with upper lobe–predominant emphysema on visual examination of the chest CT undergo perfusion scintigraphy.

So was the conclusion from NETT that LVRS was not beneficial in non-upper lobe predominant emphysema valid?

No, the conclusion drawn was that LVRS was suitable only for patients with upper lobe–predominant disease. But as we have seen retrospectively, it has been shown that there may have been problems in definition in NETT. Subsequent series over the past 25 years have shown real benefit for those with lower lobe–predominant emphysema, including those with alpha-1 antitrypsin deficiency. It is now accepted that lower lobe targets can be treated by LVR, especially in patients with alpha-1 antitrypsin deficiency [10–13]. Case Study 1 illustrates such a patient.

3.3 CASE STUDY 1: Bilobar Targets

SUMMARY

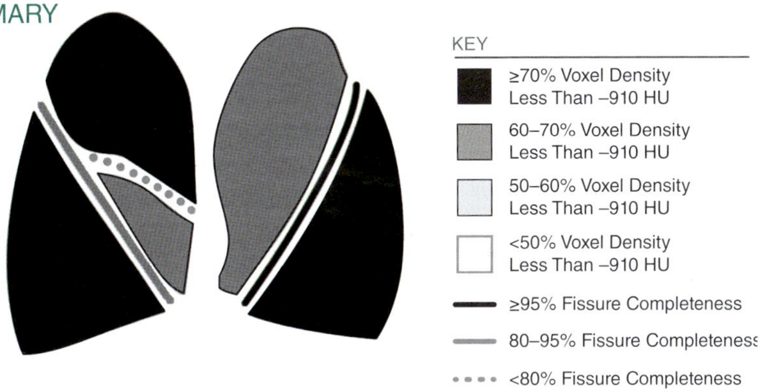

RESULTS

	RIGHT LUNG				LEFT LUNG	
	RUL	RUL + RML	RML	RLL	LUL	LLL
% Fissure Completeness	67.0	90.5	76.1	90.5	98.4	98.4
% Voxel Density Less Than –910 HU	78	75	62	81	67	72
% Voxel Density Less Than –950 HU	51	46	30	59	35	44
Inspiratory Volume (ml)	2356	3003	647	3177	2525	3156

A 67-year-old man was severely hyperinflated (as can be seen from his lung volumes above). He did not have alpha-1 anti-trypsin deficiency but was an ex-heavy smoker.

In this case, there appear to be three target lobes for LVR: the right upper, right lower and left lower lobes. In this case, the perfusion scintigraphy correlated with the emphysema severity. Fissure integrity was better on the left.

Which target would you choose and which method of LVR would you select?

As the least function was seen on the right, he underwent right LVRS with resection of diseased tissue from the both upper and lower lobes.

While left EBLVR to the lower lobe was considered, the real possibility of post-operative compensatory hyperinflation on the right guided the decision.

3.4 Risk

Which brings us back to being "bad enough to want something doing."

Very good, the last of the three Bs. But the question in selection is: can one quantify how "bad" a patient is, and who should be making that decision?

The question you're asking is: the patient or the doctor?

Of course, ideally, both parties should discuss the decision, but inevitably, the doctor will advise the patient on the basis of their understanding. Unfortunately, unless the patient or the referring doctor consults a specialist in LVR, the decision may be made on outdated or inaccurate information.

I suppose that, as LVR procedures are not commonly performed, the specialist knowledge is not widely available.

Unfortunately, that is true. Whilst the risk of LVR, particularly LVRS, may be overestimated, the best patient group for selection may not be fully appreciated.

How has NETT influenced patient selection?

The main message was that those patients with upper lobe predominant emphysema and poor exercise performance had a survival benefit, but those with better exercise tolerance had no survival benefit but did have significant improvement in quality of life [14].

Do you think that may have influenced referral practice?

It may have resulted in some referring physicians deciding that a patient may be "too good for LVR."

But aren't they just worried that the benefits may not justify the risks?

Unfortunately, the historical NETT may have given the false impression that LVRS is of high risk. The *New England Journal of Medicine* published an article quite rightly highlighting the high-risk groups before the main trial reported [15]. This sub-group of patients had both FEV_1 and DLCO below 20% of predicted and no clear heterogeneous target areas on CT. This paper was highly publicized and was, unfortunately, largely interpreted to mean that ALL patients were at high risk from LVRS.

So LVRS is not too risky?

Well, it is important not to generalize but to provide a more patient-specific risk. I prefer to use a simple risk score that we derived and tested prospectively.

Is it very complicated to calculate?

Fortunately, not at all. A prospectively validated risk score has been derived with just three parameters: absolute FEV_1, %predicted DLCO and body mass index (BMI). By allocating a value to each of these variables, the composite score separates three distinct groups: low, moderate and high based on 30-day, 90-day and 1-year mortality [16].

How risky was LVRS in the high-risk group?

In the highest-risk patients, the 30-day mortality after LVRS reached 15%, which is really too high for an elective procedure with mainly a quality-of-life benefit. However, in the low-risk group, there was only a 1% 90-day mortality.

That is surprising.

Yes, and don't forget that these "low-risk" patients may still have severe COPD, with FEV_1 of just over 700 ml/min, a DLCO of just over 20% predicted and a BMI of 19 kg/m^2.

But does the risk depend not only on the surgical selection but on the whole peri-operative care offered by an experienced team?

A very good point. Published data from experienced LVR centres in London and Belgium report a 30-day mortality below 1% [13, 17].

Are you advocating that all LVR procedures, especially LVRS, should be performed in a small number of specialist centres? It seems like a potentially risky procedure to be performed in every thoracic unit.

On the contrary, LVR is no place for heroics. It should be a high-volume, low-risk procedure in better patients who stand to get more benefit. It should not be restricted to patients too old for transplantation in those specialized centres. I am concerned that both forms of LVR procedure may be interpreted as "lifesaving."

What do you think is wrong with that idea? So, can the patient be too unwell for LVR? Isn't that a good use of LVR, particularly as a lung transplant may not be a realistic option for many more elderly patients?

While experienced centres with lung transplant experience may be ideally suited to treating these very borderline patients, I believe that the real benefits of LVR lie in patients at the better end of the spectrum.

You mean lower-risk but still symptomatic people.

Yes, I think that the ideal place for LVR is in the typical middle-aged patient who may be struggling to keep their job due to breathlessness on minimal exertion or may be threatened with having to move from their second-floor home as they struggle up the stairs.

These cases are quite common, I guess.

They are, but they are probably not considered for LVR in many centres for the reasons above.

Doesn't that put the newer, less experienced centres in a difficult situation?

Absolutely, the irony is that concentrating on the higher risk, more disabled patients for LVR will result in potentially more postoperative complications and longer hospital stays. As shown in Figure 3.6, these factors will put pressure on these centres just starting out on an LVR programme to start with higher-risk patients whose more complicated recovery may dissuade further referrals, which may even lead to premature termination of the service.

So, a larger number of more straightforward, patients of better performance is the ideal way to begin an LVR service?

That is exactly the message to spread amongst referring physicians and why a fledgling service should cast its net wide into the better end of the spectrum and be very selective in patient selection (Figure 3.7). By increasing the upper limits of referral criteria and by filtering out those

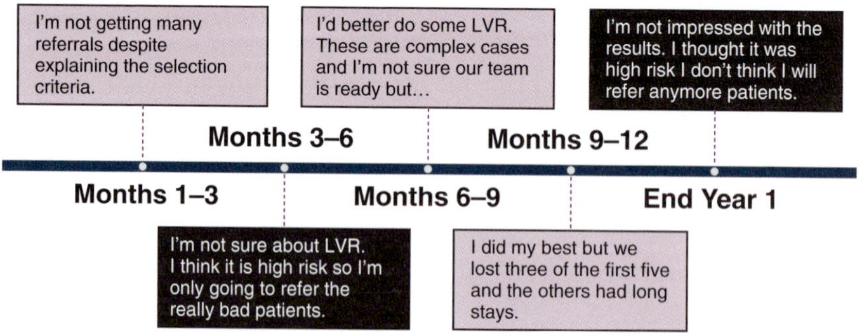

Figure 3.6 The timeline of an LVR service destined to fail.

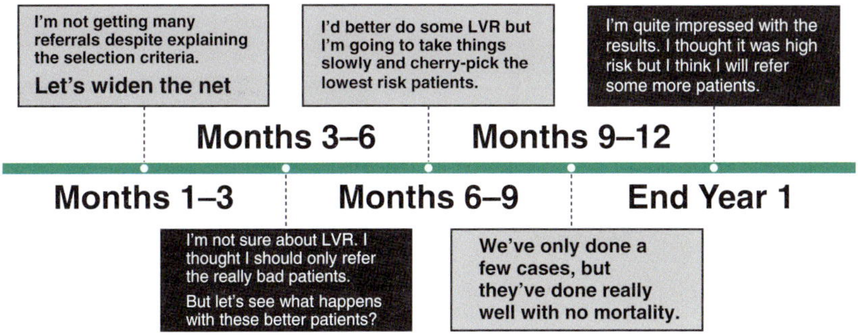

Figure 3.7 The timeline of an LVR service destined to succeed.

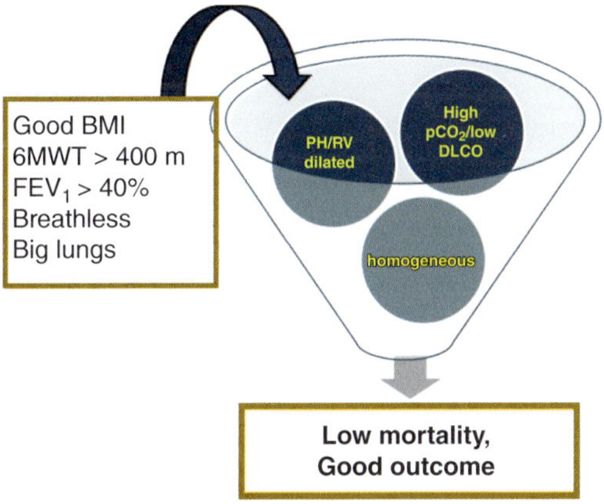

Figure 3.8 The principles of a successful selection process for LVR.

at the lower end of the spectrum, the LVR pathway is strengthened (Figure 3.8).

But going back to what we said previously, aren't the referring physicians going to say that some of these patients are too good for LVR?

There is evidence that severely hyperinflated patients with a heterogeneous morphology can be considered for lung volume reduction surgery even if they are above the upper limit criteria for FEV_1 and 6-minute walk distance (6MWD). Of course, the postoperative risk is minimal, but they still observe significant clinical benefits [18].

And what is the outcome for the higher-risk patients?

Those patients who are confined to a wheelchair and on long-term oxygen therapy or non-invasive ventilation should be managed in more

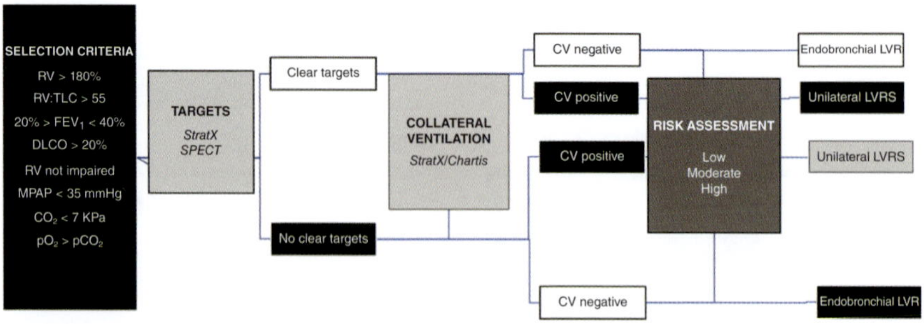

Figure 3.9 The four-stage LVR selection process.

experienced centres until their local centre has achieved consistently good results.

So, can you summarize the LVR selection process?

I think it is easiest to view it as a four-stage process (Figure 3.9). The first stage is to establish the cardiorespiratory selection data regarding lung volumes, gas exchange and cardiac function. The second stage surrounds target selection by correlating anatomical and physiological images. Then, as we shall see in later chapters, the decision regarding which method of LVR is most suitable can be made by the LVR MDT. Finally, the individualized risk of the proposed procedure can be calculated and discussed with the patient.

3.5 Conclusions

I suggest that to simplify the selection process for LVR, one considers the 3Bs and 4Gs.

The 3Bs: big lungs, breathless and bad enough to want something done. So, a patient who is so breathless from their hyperinflation that they are prepared to take the risk of intervention to improve their quality (not primarily quantity) of life.

The 4Gs: good gases, good heart, good legs and good targets. This means avoiding severe hypercapnia and pulmonary hypertension with right ventricular dysfunction. It implies that the patient has received pulmonary rehabilitation and attained their optimal exercise capacity. Finally, it acknowledges that the best outcomes are obtained in those with the most defined areas of emphysematous, functionless lungs.

The selection spectrum has two extremes, and the novice programme should begin at the better end in order to establish the pathway and only then slowly move toward the more complex end as experience grows.

References

1 Fumat R, Dupuis M, Mallah S, Heluain V, Favard F, Simonneau Y, et al. Impact of bronchoscopic lung volume reduction with endobronchial valves on dynamic hyperinflation: Results from the PIERCE study. Respirology. 2023;28(6):525–532.
2 Wisser W, Klepetko W, Senbaklavaci O, Wanke T, Gruber E, Tschernko E, et al. Chronic hypercapnia should not exclude patients from lung volume reduction surgery. Eur J Cardiothorac Surg. 1998;14:107–112.
3 Kessler R, Oswald-Mammosser M. Does lung volume reduction surgery compromise the pulmonary circulation? Am J Respir Crit Care Med. 1999; 160(4):1429–1430.
4 Caviezel C, Aruldas C, Franzen D, Ulrich S, Inci I, Schneiter D, et al. Lung volume reduction surgery in selected patients with emphysema and pulmonary hypertension. Eur J Cardiothorac Surg. 2018;54:565–571.
5 Eberhardt R, Gerovasili V, Kontogianni K, Gompelmann D, Ehlken N, Herth FJ, et al. Endoscopic lung volume reduction with endobronchial valves in patients with severe emphysema and established pulmonary hypertension. Respiration. 2015;89(1):41–48.
6 Tee VST, Nguyen P, Jersmann H, Grosser D, Crouch B, Lorraine B, et al. Use of ventilation-perfusion single-photon emission computed tomography to select the target lobe for endobronchial valve lung volume reduction. Respiration. 2021;100(9):886–897.
7 Hartman JE, Roodenburg SA, van Dijk M, Koster TD, Klooster K, Slebos DJ. Response to endobronchial valve treatment: it's all about the target lobe. ERJ Open Res. 2023;9(4):00155–2023.
8 Chandra D, Lipson DA, Hoffman EA, Hansen-Flaschen J, Sciurba FC, Decamp MM, et al. Perfusion scintigraphy and patient selection for lung volume reduction surgery. Am J Respir Crit Care Med. 2010;182(7):937–946.
9 Wang Z, Gu S, Leader JK, Kundu S, Tedrow JR, Sciurba FC, et al. Optimal threshold in CT quantification of emphysema. Eur Radiol. 2013;23(4):975–984.
10 Perikleous P, Sharkey A, Oey I, Bilancia R, Tenconi S, Rathinam S, et al. Long-term survival and symptomatic relief in lower lobe lung volume reduction surgery. Eur J Cardiothorac Surg. 2017;52(5):982–988.
11 Zahid I, Sharif S, Routledge T, Scarci M. Is lung volume reduction surgery effective in the treatment of advanced emphysema? Interact Cardiovasc Thorac Surg. 2011;12(3):480–486.

12 Naunheim KS, Wood DE, Mohsenifar Z, Sternberg AL, Criner GJ, DeCamp MM, et al. Long-term follow-up of patients receiving lung-volume-reduction surgery versus medical therapy for severe emphysema by the National Emphysema Treatment Trial Research Group. Ann Thorac Surg. 2006;82(2):431–443.

13 Ceulemans LJ, Vandervelde CM, Everaerts S, Dooms C, Geysen H, Fontaine M, et al. Low mortality and favourable outcome in lung volume reduction surgery for different emphysema morphologies. Eur Respir J. 2025;65:2501133.

14 Fishman A, Martinez F, Naunheim K, Piantadosi S, Wise R, Ries A, et al. A randomized trial comparing lung-volume-reduction surgery with medical therapy for severe emphysema. N Engl J Med. 2003;348:2059–2073.

15 National Emphysema Treatment Trial Research Group, Fishman A, Fessler H, Martinez F, McKenna RJ Jr, Naunheim K, et al. Patients at high risk of death after lung-volume-reduction surgery. N Engl J Med. 2001;345(15):1075–1083.

16 Greening NJ, Vaughan P, Oey I, Steiner MC, Morgan MD, Rathinam S, et al. Individualised risk in patients undergoing lung volume reduction surgery: the Glenfield BFG score. Eur Respir J. 2017;49(6):1601766.

17 Clark SJ, Zoumot Z, Bamsey O, Polkey MI, Dusmet M, Lim E, et al. Surgical approaches for lung volume reduction in emphysema. Clin Med (Lond). 2014;14(2):122–127.

18 Vandervelde CM, Everaerts S, Weder W, Dooms C, Slebos DJ, Janssens W, et al. Widening the selection criteria for lung volume reduction surgery. Eur Respir J. 2025;65(1):2400829.

4

Technique: Lung Volume Reduction Surgery

4.1 Approach

Junior lung volume reduction surgeon (LVRS): Are we agreed on which is the best way to approach lung volume reduction surgery?

Senior LVR surgeon: Well (as we discussed in Chapter 2) the original description by Brantigan involved bilateral thoracotomy, but Cooper promoted a median sternotomy approach to facilitate bilateral one-stage LVRS.

Presumably, minimally invasive surgery has now become the approach of choice.

Yes, the reinvention of LVRS coincided with the advent of video-assisted thoracic surgery (VATS), which was particularly attractive in these patients with poor lung function. Non-randomized comparisons showed improved outcomes from VATS due to reduced postoperative morbidity [1].

Were there any drawbacks to the use of VATS?

When we opened the sternum, it was fairly straightforward to assess the most hyperinflated parts of the lung by manual palpation. However, using VATS, the lung remained inflated even when non-ventilating for a few minutes. It is imperative that the double-lumen tube is correctly sited; thus, the experience of the anaesthetist was of paramount importance.

I understand that some surgeons have attempted LVRS without endotracheal intubation.

Yes, there is a group of pioneers in Rome who have attempted unilateral, uniportal LVRS without muscle paralysis and endotracheal intubation. However, I think it is an exaggeration to call this "awake" surgery [2].

The patients are heavily sedated with intravenous propofol and remifentanil and breathe through a laryngeal mask to protect their airway. As one might expect, they only maintain low tidal volume spontaneous ventilation and thus require the Anaesthetist to intermittently use manually assisted ventilation to keep oxygen saturation up and the end-tidal carbon dioxide levels down.

It sounds like there may be some practical intraoperative problems.

Yes, in my experience, the drawback is reduced visibility due to lung expansion and the possibility of intermittent coughing.

Is there any way around this problem?

In my experience, a good manoeuvre is to deliberately puncture the target area to expedite deflation. The concern that this would create a large air leak and destabilize the patient has not been a problem, possibly because these most damaged areas are poorly ventilated anyway. Some also advocate using local anaesthetic around the vagus nerve to dampen the cough mechanism, but this effect may hamper postoperative recovery.

So, is spontaneous ventilation a good development?

I would not recommend it as the patient has to be quite heavily sedated and therefore is relatively hypoventilating. Unless the operation is very quick, then hypercapnia can be a problem and ironically, may require a period of assisted ventilation to facilitate recovery. The enthusiasts report a minor reduction in hospital stay of 1–2 days, but it does not appear to have extended their selection criteria into higher-risk cases. I would have thought that the best use of the spontaneous ventilation method would be to potentially facilitate a smoother recovery from the procedure.

How much of a problem are pleural adhesions?

Occasionally, particularly if there was a history of previous pneumonia or pneumothorax. But they are difficult to predict yet fairly easy to mobilize with electrocautery or latterly other energy devices. So, there is a balance to be struck between sufficient adhesiolysis to give adequate exposure and excessive mobilization leading to persistent air leak.

The big decision is whether you would convert to thoracotomy to deal with dense adhesions or would you abandon the procedure?

Great question. I have only encountered this once in over 500 LVRS procedures when I bailed out. I think a lot of the risk is from the general anaesthesia itself, so once committed, just continue. The caveat to that

statement is that I would only proceed with open LVRS if I thought that good analgesia could be obtained and the patient was at the lower end of the risk spectrum and more able to deal with the complications from post-operative pneumonia.

Has the advent of robotic-assisted thoracic surgery (RATS) impacted LVRS?

The technique is still in its infancy, but I have found several advantages in the use of RATS. Firstly, the capnothorax does help to collapse the lung, but also helps to differentiate those areas that are most emphysematous, which are slower to collapse. Secondly, it is possible to use an intravenous injection of indocyanine green (ICG) and the near infrared thoracoscopic application [3] to identify differential perfusion in the target lobe in vivo (Figure 4.1a,b). The technique needs some refinement (with timing and dosage), but it sometimes suggests that areas are of better perfusion than expected and can be preserved. This technique is now available to use with VATS. Finally, I find the RATS instruments to be beneficial, with the "intelligent" stapling devices leading to better thickness selection. The staplers will not fire if the tissue is too thick and not compressed; they also fire slowly to maximize the efficiency of the instrument. When using VATS, the staplers may be fired too quickly or excessive manual force may be applied to overcome a tissue thickness mismatch.

Robotic-assisted lung volume reduction surgery. Demarcation between relatively well-perfused lung tissue (green) from more functionless emphysematous lung demonstrated under near infrared thoracoscopy following intravenous indocyanine green injection.

Are there any practical advantages in terms of outcome?

My initial impressions are that more targeted resection with improved stapling may lead to reduced postoperative air leak.

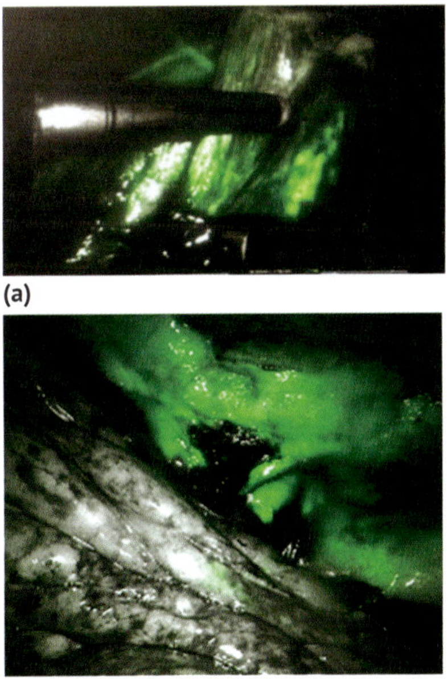

(a)

(b)

Figure 4.1 **(a, b)** Robotic-assisted lung volume reduction surgery.

4.2 Operative Technique

Many surgeons have the impression that LVRS is a relatively simple operation of just "a few wedge resections." Don't you think they are underestimating the technical requirements?

Definitely. It can be easy to make a few wrong moves and end up with a large apical space and persistent air leak with worsening subcutaneous emphysema. The patient may not recover from a simple intraoperative mistake. Thus, accuracy is paramount.

What would you say are the main surgical principles in LVRS?

Firstly, do no harm. LVRS is effectively trying to remodel "candy floss." Manipulation and division of the destroyed emphysematous lung tissue are prone to parenchymal damage and air leak. So, a "minimal touch" technique, avoiding pointed or heavy metallic instruments, is a starting point [4].

And how much lung should be resected?

The question that has never been convincingly answered in 30 years of LVRS. There have been attempts to quantify the extent of LVRS by the weight of the specimen removed. It was shown that there was an association between the weight of lung resected and the improvement in forced expiratory volume in one second (FEV_1), but there was considerable variability in the response, and there was no apparent relationship between the amount of tissue resected and overall postoperative survival [5].

So, the surgery remains more of an art than a science.

In principle, sufficient lung should be removed to actually obtain significant "volume reduction" and reduce hyperinflation, but not so much that too much functioning lung is removed or a large, irregular remaining pleural space is left. Ideally, guided by preoperative and now intraoperative imaging, the lung should be remodelled so that its contours will match the reconfigured chest wall. As Brantigan stated, "to reshape the target lobe to its premorbid shape in expiration "whilst also minimizing the number of staple lines."

Do you use any anatomical landmarks or stapling strategies?

For the right upper lobe, I resect down to the level of the azygos vein (Figure 4.2a,b) and on the left down to the level of the aortic arch. For lower lobe LVRS, it is more difficult as the level of the inferior pulmonary

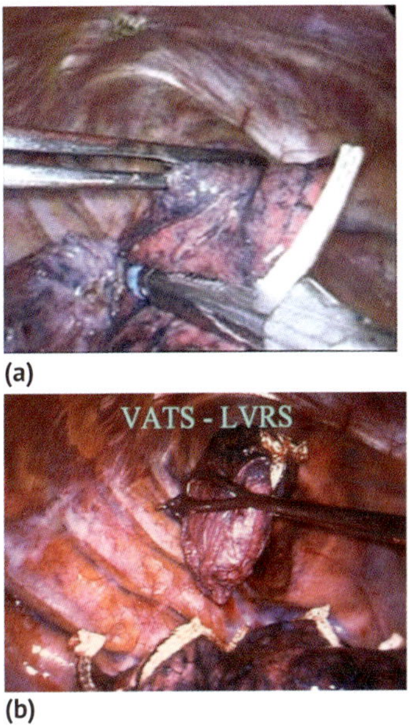

Figure 4.2 **(a, b)** Operative extent of resection in the right upper lobe LVRS.

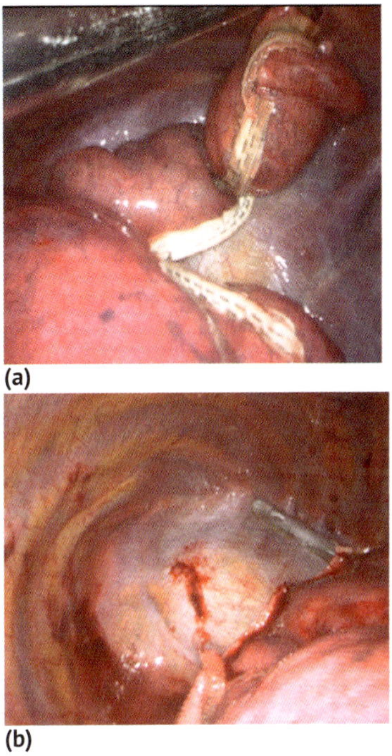

Figure 4.3 **(a, b)** Operative extent of resection in the left lower lobe LVRS.

vein is too high and leaves too much potential pleural space. In general, I would aim to remove up to 40% of the target lobe volume on initial inspection (Figure 4.3a,b).

Regarding the stapling strategies, there are several versions of "a few wedge resections." The original technique of Cooper and the American surgeons in the 1990s was basically an apical "crescent" resection of the upper lobe apex (Figure 4.4a,b). I prefer the "horseshoe" resection to give a more three-dimensional volume reduction and potentially less apical residual space (Figure 4.5a,b).

The margin of resection continues to be a subjective assessment by the surgeon. Some will insufflate air into the target lobe just prior to resection to observe where the lung is slowest to deflate [4] or the use of ICG and near infrared thoracoscopy, as we have mentioned, to identify the margin by fluorescence shows promise [3].

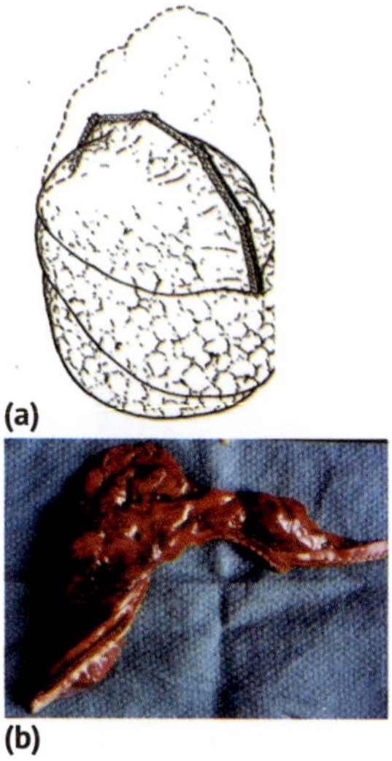

Figure 4.4 **(a, b)** The apical resection technique.

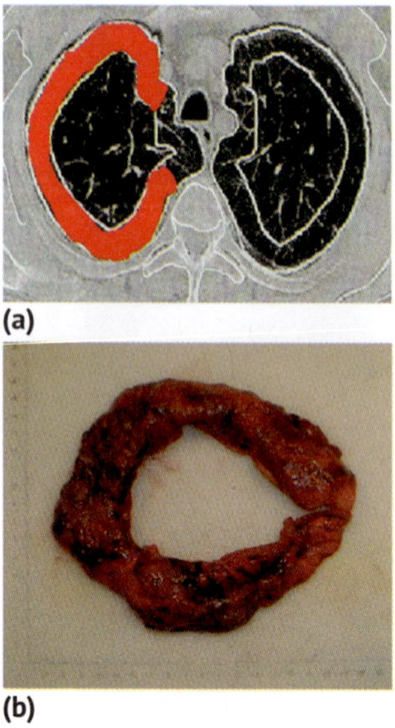

Figure 4.5 **(a, b)** The resection technique.

What other measures can be taken to reduce postoperative air leak? Do you reinforce the staple lines?

I have tried many materials (bovine pericardium, PTFE, vicryl and synthetic sealants) to buttress the staple lines without any significant benefit, and they are not without complications, including expectoration of the buttress or staples [6] or pseudotumour formation due to the inflammatory reaction [7].

How on Earth does that happen?

I cannot imagine the staples migrating retrogradely through the airways! I suggest that the inflammation around a staple line may result in a small fistula into a major airway. Although it should be noted that these events are rare and are not associated with pneumothorax or any significant morbidity.

I understand that some surgeons have significantly modified their technique to reduce air leak.

That is correct. The non-resectional technique has been proposed involving either simply removing the blade from the stapler or by in-folding or "plicating" the target lung tissue before stapling [8, 9].

This sounds like a more complicated procedure. Is it worth it?

Well, on the occasions I have returned to reoperate for this complication, the leak has NOT been from the staple line but rather from another diseased part of either the target or non-target lobe, presumably resulting from redistribution of ventilation. Thus, I prefer to apply a tissue adhesive over the area adjacent to the staple line at the end of the procedure.

Would you ever consider a lobectomy in these situations?

A very interesting question. Many surgeons will perform a lobectomy if they are concerned about the quality of the remaining target lobe after LVRS.

So, why not?

Firstly, LVRS is a compromise between reducing hyperinflation but retaining function. So, there may be occasions when the target lobe has very little function and lobectomy may be the best approach providing the fissure can be dissected safely (more on that later). The most common scenario would be in a lower lobe target in a patient with alpha-1 antitrypsin deficiency.

Secondly, removing a large lobe may result in a size mismatch between the residual lung and the thoracic cage, thus perpetuating a postoperative air leak.

We can discuss the management of postoperative air leaks later, but the best management is prevention, and the best time is at the end of the operation. Before closing the wounds, just test the lung under water in reinflation and deal with any obvious leaks with more stapling at that time. The anaesthetist may be able to indicate a very large air leak when double lung ventilation is resumed, so listen to their advice.

4.3 Perioperative Care

What are the important messages to convey to your anaesthetist?

Perhaps most importantly, the fact that patients do very well after LVRS if carefully selected, and they should not fear the worst.

Do they need to book an intensive care bed for the patient postoperatively?

That is a moot point! With experience, the need for a pre-booked critical care bed seems superfluous, but in the first few cases, this may act as added reassurance. The key point is that the surgery should improve lung

function and offset any immediate side effects of the incisions or general anaesthesia.

Would a short period of elective mechanical ventilation not facilitate a smoother recovery from the operation?

In practice, this is very difficult as positive pressure ventilation will not only increase any potential air leak from the operated lung but also run the risk of air trapping and hyperinflation in the non-operated lung.

So, what are the key steps to avoid the need for postoperative critical care?

Simply, avoid pain and respiratory depression.

Which means avoid opiates?

Absolutely! I would advocate pre-emptive regional analgesia. Depending on the available expertise, I would favour epidural analgesia, but an intraoperative paravertebral/intercostal local anaesthetic block may be preferred as soon as the camera is in the chest. Some colleagues find that intraoperative cryoanalgesia of several intercostal nerves above and below the incisions is effective. I would also add that multiport VATS or RATS should be performed by no more than three small incisions in the same intercostal space. I have no experience with uniportal LVRS, but access must be adequate to allow remodelling of the lung with adequate tissue removal.

Obviously, I must ask about drain management, as this can impact postoperative pain.

I think the most important lessons I have learned are: (1) it is easier to remove a drain than insert another postoperatively, and (2) the remaining lung does not rapidly expand to fill the space after optimal volume reduction.

So, from that, I assume the use of two drains, but not on suction.

Correct, inadequate drainage can potentiate the complication of subcutaneous emphysema, and inappropriate use of suction can lead to a pressure-dependent air leak and the complications of long-term drainage.

And the lack of suction or the use of flutter valve bags will facilitate postoperative mobilization.

Indeed, "bed is bad" for the LVRS patient. Early intermittent ambulation interspersed with rest in the sitting (not supine) position is the mantra. This is when a period of preoperative education on the pulmonary rehabilitation programme will pay dividends.

What are your thoughts about a specific medication for an LVRS patient?

I would have a low threshold for the use of oral steroids with antibiotic cover at the earliest suspicion of an exacerbation of the underlying COPD. This can be empirical or based on any evidence that the patient has characteristics of the asthma-COPD overlap phenotype. Of course, nebulized bronchodilators and anti-thromboembolism precautions are mandatory.

4.4 Controversies

All sounds very logical, but there is one point that I need to clarify. I cannot understand why you would want to deviate from the original technique of one-stage bilateral LVRS, which was shown to be beneficial by Brantigan, Cooper and in the NETT?

Ah, the "Tortoise and the Hare" debate! One-stage bilateral versus staged unilateral.

Exactly, but I would favour surgical common sense over an ancient fable!

I would respectfully reflect that those surgical descriptions you refer to belong to the last century. Time has moved on, and there is an alternative thought process. Rather than one great, heroic intervention, I would prefer a more stealthy, cautious approach. The tortoise overtook the hare. Don't forget [10].

But don't we know that the benefits in lung function are significantly greater after bilateral than unilateral LVRS?

We do, but they also decline at a faster rate.

In one of the original series, the short-term improvement in FEV_1 was 390 ml for bilateral LVRS and 250 ml for unilateral LVRS. However, the long-term rate of decline in FEV_1 was greatest for bilateral staple LVRS procedures as well: 255 ml/yr for bilateral vs 107 ml/yr for unilateral LVRS. There was a relationship between the magnitude of short-term incremental improvement and the rate of deterioration in FEV_1 [11].

And the risks are no greater with one-stage bilateral LVRS.

I agree that the risk of LVRS should not depend on the approach, but significant bilateral air leaks can be dangerous and may prolong the postoperative stay. We switched from routine bilateral LVRS to a staged unilateral approach, as there was no significant benefit in quality of life, but there was increased morbidity and mortality from operating on both lungs at the same operation [12], findings which are still reported [13].

But leaving a native severely emphysematous contralateral lung runs the risk of compensatory hyperinflation or pneumothorax.

That is true, but quite a rare occurrence. So, I would be cautious in the case of severe bilateral emphysema and advocate a mandated second unilateral operation within a few weeks once the patient has recovered from the first.

So, you would not make a plan for the second unilateral operation anyway once recovery from the first had been achieved, as has been suggested [14, 15]?

No, I prefer to leave the decision in the hands of the patient. The procedure is intended to lead to an improvement in quality of life. This is subjective and determined by the patient. If you fix the time interval to 3–6 months, then either the patient is doing really well and therefore can only experience a fall in quality of life, or they are no better than preoperatively, so further LVR is unlikely to help, and they are symptomatic for some other reason than hyperinflation.

I can see that, but I would be worried that patients may be lost to follow-up or wait too long and become unsuitable for the second operation. They would have therefore missed out on the potential greater benefit of bilateral LVRS.

That may happen to a minority, but in the majority, they can benefit from a second "boost" of LVR. Initial claims that bilateral LVRS resulted in greater long-term survival [16] were probably misleading due to selection bias.

In a subgroup analysis of the last 45 patients assessed for the second-stage LVR in our patient-directed staged protocol, 31% were not suitable at reassessment due to disease progression. This was apparent as deterioration in diffusion capacity (although over 3 years since their first stage), significant pulmonary hypertension, increasing infective complications from which two died during reassessment, loss of a clear target area, and finally, one patient proceeded to lung transplantation [17].

So, one in three missed out on the benefits of bilateral LVRS?

The contrary argument is this: in our experience, over 250 patients, we found that only one in four requested a second operation, and yet the improvements in quality-of-life measures were significantly greater in the unilateral/staged unilateral group than the one-stage bilateral group and remained so for up to nearly a decade [17].

Is it possible to combine LVRS and EBLVR in a sequential fashion?

Certainly, there have been several reports, including our own experience, of operating after a previous EBLVR. LVRS has been successfully used as a salvage after EBLVR. It may be used on the previous target lobe, which has failed to collapse, or it can be used to treat progressive emphysema or accelerated compensatory hyperinflation in non-target lobes. Some have found the results to be better for primary failure than secondary deterioration due to worsening disease [18].

Is it also possible to insert valves after LVRS?

More rarely, endobronchial valves have been placed into a target lobe that has hyperinflated after previous LVRS. But in these cases, LVRS was performed before the advent of regular EBLVR, and fortuitously, no collateral ventilation was present. The distortion of the anatomy can create a challenging situation in the placement of valves in the apical upper lobe segments [17].

So, is this a very limited option?

Well, not necessarily.

Go on.

We will discuss the use of surgical division of the incomplete interlobar fissure in later chapters. But consider the potential benefits of adding fissure division routinely to unilateral LVRS. This would facilitate a secondary procedure of EBLVR when and if the target lobe reinflates years after LVRS. This could be viewed as prophylactic fissure division to facilitate second-stage EBLVR by eliminating the possibility of collateral ventilation.

Yes, that sounds very sensible if the risk of increased air leak was justifiable, and I would be concerned about adding extra dissection and more staple lines.

We have also presented some initial data that suggest that the outcome of LVRS, as measured by improvement in FEV_1, correlates with increased fissure integrity. So, prophylactic fissure division may improve the initial outcome of the procedure [19].

How do you explain that finding?

Interestingly, the improvement was independently related to fissure integrity (not related to any of the other selection criteria) and therefore presumably to the presence of collateral channels of Martin. One could hypothesize that if resistance through these channels was less than that of the normal airways in the emphysematous lung. Improved ventilation

of the target lobe after LVRS may encourage translobar ventilation of the non-target lobe, resulting in increased hyperinflation to the detriment of the eventual outcome of volume reduction.

That is an interesting hypothesis that merits further research.

I agree, but nevertheless, I would like to reiterate that repeated intervention can spread out the overall benefit of LVR and keep the patients' quality of life "above baseline" for longer. After all, if one performs standard bilateral LVRS, where do you go next?

Lung transplantation?

Quite...

4.5 Conclusions

Let us work through an illustrative case study to summarize our statements.

4.5.1 CASE STUDY: Perioperative Management of an LVRS Case

This 67-year-old male is breathless, has big lungs (RV 280% predicted) and is bad enough to want intervention.

He has COPD (FEV_1 28% predicted) but has an acceptable risk profile as his diffusion capacity is 35% predicted, and he has no evidence of right heart dysfunction and is normocapnic.

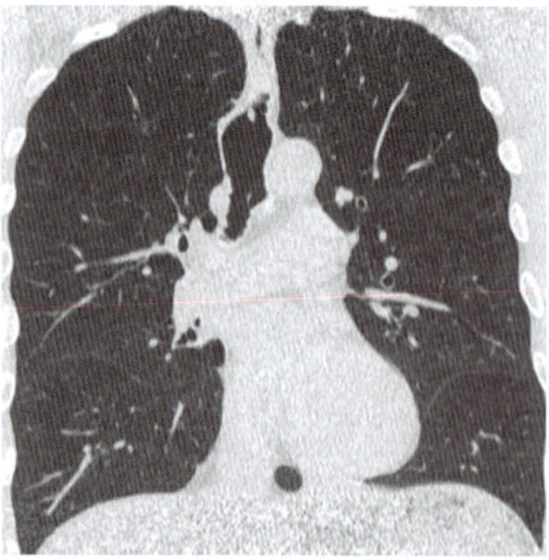

SUMMARY

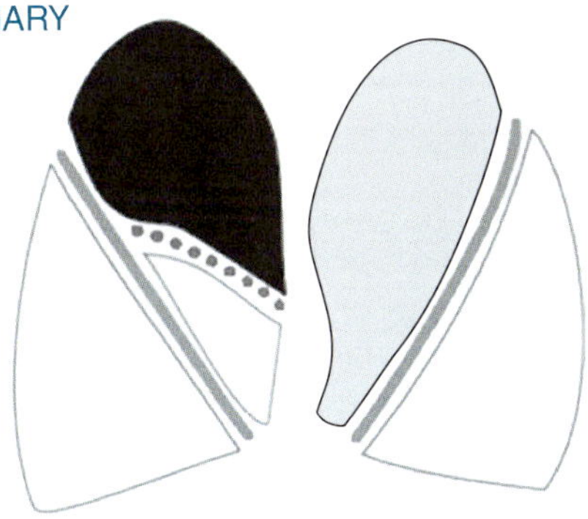

KEY

- ≥70% Voxel Density Less Than −910 HU
- 60–70% Voxel Density Less Than −910 HU
- 50–60% Voxel Density Less Than −910 HU
- <50% Voxel Density Less Than −910 HU
- ≥95% Fissure Completeness
- 80–95% Fissure Completeness
- <80% Fissure Completeness

RESULTS

	RIGHT LUNG				LEFT LUNG	
	RUL	RUL + RML	RML	RLL	LUL	LLL
% Fissure Completeness	57.0	87.4	62.8	87.4	86.6	86.6
% Voxel Density Less Than −910 HU	71	67	49	43	52	27
% Voxel Density Less Than −950 HU	53	48	25	20	25	12
Inspiratory Volume (ml)	2493	2989	496	1347	2428	1221

His CT imaging with software analysis (StratX) demonstrates bilateral upper lobe targets with the highest severity (over 50% density <−950 HU) in the right upper lobe and the largest volume in the right upper and middle lobes.

The interlobar fissures are of borderline integrity (<90% open) for consideration of endobronchial LVR, but high enough to consider testing for collateral ventilation and attempt EBLVR.

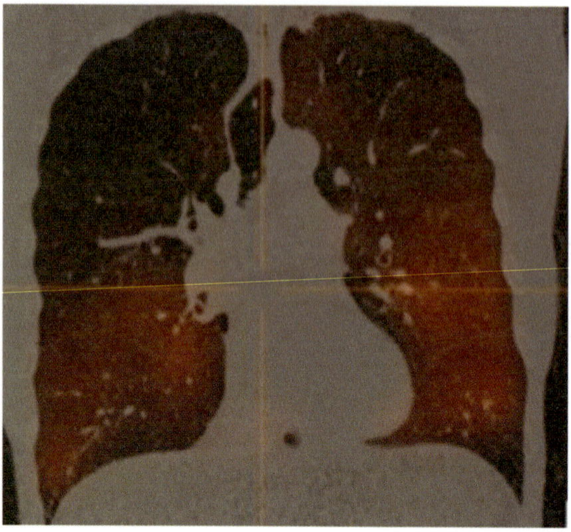

His SPECT scan correlates with the CT analysis, confirming the right upper lobe to be clearly the most functionless target.

It would be reasonable to discuss the option of RIGHT EBLVR, but this would require an initial Chartis® assessment.

If this was positive for collateral ventilation on the RIGHT major fissure but negative on the LEFT, which option would you choose?

I would be concerned about compensatory hyperinflation of the RIGHT upper lobe if the LEFT upper lobe were to be collapsed together with the greater loss of function. So, I would go for the RIGHT LVRS of the upper and possibly the middle lobe.

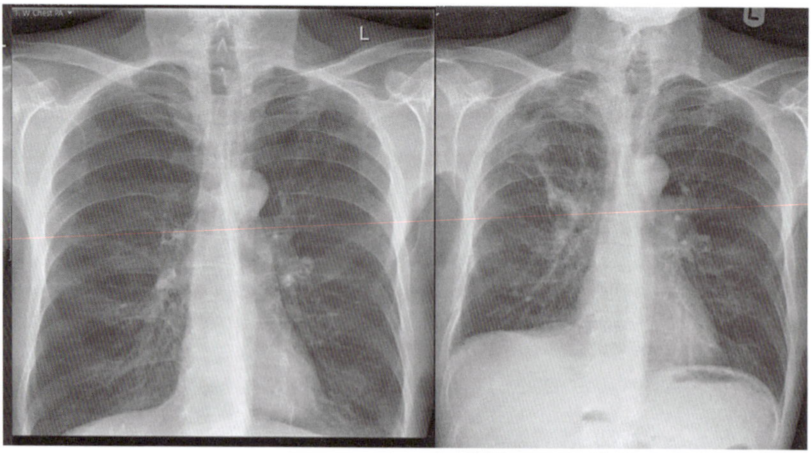

The patient underwent right upper lobe LVRS with excellent restoration of diaphragmatic contour *bilaterally* and significant symptomatic improvement.

References

1 Brenner M, Yusen R, McKenna R Jr, Sciurba F, Gelb AF, Fischel R, et al. Lung volume reduction surgery for emphysema. Chest. 1996;110(1):205–218. https://doi.org/10.1378/chest.110.1.205

2 Pompeo E, Rogliani P, Tacconi F, Dauri M, Saltini C, Novelli G, et al. Randomized comparison of awake nonresectional versus nonawake resectional lung volume reduction surgery. J Thorac Cardiovasc Surg. 2012;143(1):47–54, 54.e1.

3 Li H, Zhou J, Chi C, Mao Y, Yang F, Tian J, et al. Clinical application of near-infrared thoracoscope with indocyanine green in video-assisted thoracoscopic bullectomy. J Thorac Dis. 2016;8(7):1841–1845.

4 Ceulemans LJ, Vandervelde CM, Everaerts S, Dooms C, Geysen H, Fontaine M, et al. Low mortality and favourable outcome in lung volume reduction surgery for different emphysema morphologies. Eur Respir J. 2025;65:2501133.

5 Brenner M, McKenna RJ Jr, Chen JC, Serna DL, Powell LL, Gelb AF, et al. Relationship between amount of lung resected and outcome after lung volume reduction surgery. Ann Thorac Surg. 2000;69(2):388–393.

6 Oey I, Waller DA. Metalloptysis: a late complication of lung volume reduction surgery. Ann Thorac Surg. 2001;71(5):1694–1695.

7 Oey IF, Jeyapalan K, Entwisle JJ, Waller DA. Pseudo tumours of the lung after lung volume reduction surgery. Ann Thorac Surg. 2004;77(3):1094–1096.

8 Swanson SJ, Mentzer SJ, DeCamp MM, Bueno R, Richard WG, Ingenito EP, et al. No-cut thoracoscopic lung plication: a new technique for lung volume reduction surgery. J Am Coll Surg. 1997;185:25–32.

9 Pompeo E, Elkhouly A, Rogliani P, Dauri M, Peer M, Sergiacomi G, et al. Quasilobar minimalist lung volume reduction surgery. Eur J Cardiothorac Surg. 2021;60(3):598–606.

10 Aesop's Fables. Fable 226. 2020 Sep 23. https://aesopsfables.org/

11 Brenner M, McKenna RJ Jr, Gelb AF, Fischel RJ, Wilson A. Rate of FEV1 change following lung volume reduction surgery. Chest. 1998;113:652–659.

12 Oey IF, Waller DA, Bal S, Singh SJ, Spyt TJ, Morgan MD. Lung volume reduction surgery – a comparison of the long-term outcome of unilateral vs. bilateral approaches. Eur J Cardiothorac Surg. 2002;22(4):610–614.

13 Castillo-Larios R, Yu Lee-Mateus A, Hernandez-Rojas D, Pulipaka P, Thomas M, Jacob S, El-Sayed Ahmed MM, Fernandez-Bussy S, Abia-Trujillo D, Makey IA.

Outcomes of lung volume reduction surgery for emphysema: unilateral and bilateral. J Thorac Dis. 2024;16(10):6406–6416.

14 Soon SY, Saidi G, Ong ML, Syed A, Codispoti M, Walker WS. Sequential VATS lung volume reduction surgery: prolongation of benefits derived after the initial operation. Eur J Cardiothorac Surg. 2003;24(1):149–153.

15 Pompeo E, Mineo TC, Pulmonary Emphysema Research Group. Long-term outcome of staged versus one-stage bilateral thoracoscopic reduction pneumoplasty. Eur J Cardiothorac Surg. 2002;21(4):627–633.

16 Serna DL, Brenner M, Osann KE, McKenna RJ Jr, Chen JC, Fischel RJ, et al. Survival after unilateral versus bilateral lung volume reduction surgery for emphysema. J Thorac Cardiovasc Surg. 1999;118(6):1101–1109.

17 Oey I, Steiner M, Morgan M, Waller D. Patient-directed volume reduction for emphysema: sequential surgical and endobronchial techniques. Ann Thorac Surg. 2021;112(1):295–301.

18 Caviezel C, Guglielmetti LC, Ladan M, Hansen HJ, Perch M, Schneiter D, et al. Lung volume reduction surgery as salvage procedure after previous use of endobronchial valves. Interact Cardiovasc Thorac Surg. 2021;32(2):263–269.

19 Shanahan B. Novel uses of quantitative CT software in lung volume reduction. O-072, 32nd Annual Meeting of the European Society of Thoracic Surgeons; 2024, Barcelona.

5

Technique: Endobronchial Lung Volume Reduction

Trainee: There do seem to be many methods that have been attempted to achieve lung volume reduction (LVR) via the bronchoscope rather than by surgery. Is there a way of grouping them to assess their relative merits?

Trainer: Yes, we can divide them by the proposed method of obtaining LVR. The first couple of methods are attempts to mechanically combat the expiratory airways collapse associated with emphysema.

5.1 Airway Bypass

The technique involves bronchoscopic creation of new artificial, extra-anatomical communications through bronchial walls into the parenchyma of emphysematous lung tissue. These bypass channels are then held open by the insertion of small stents (Figure 5.1).

The intent was to relieve the gas trapping by increasing both the rate and volume of air expelled during forced expiration [1]. They were theoretically ideal for patients without clear target areas.

How was this method evaluated?

A randomized, double-blind, sham-controlled trial, EASE, of 315 patients showed no significant improvement in lung function or dyspnoea score [2].

What were the problems?

These stents became blocked with either mucus plugs or in the longer-term granulation tissue. These complications made the stents non-functional and increased the incidence of respiratory infection and acute exacerbations of the underlying chronic obstructive pulmonary disease (COPD).

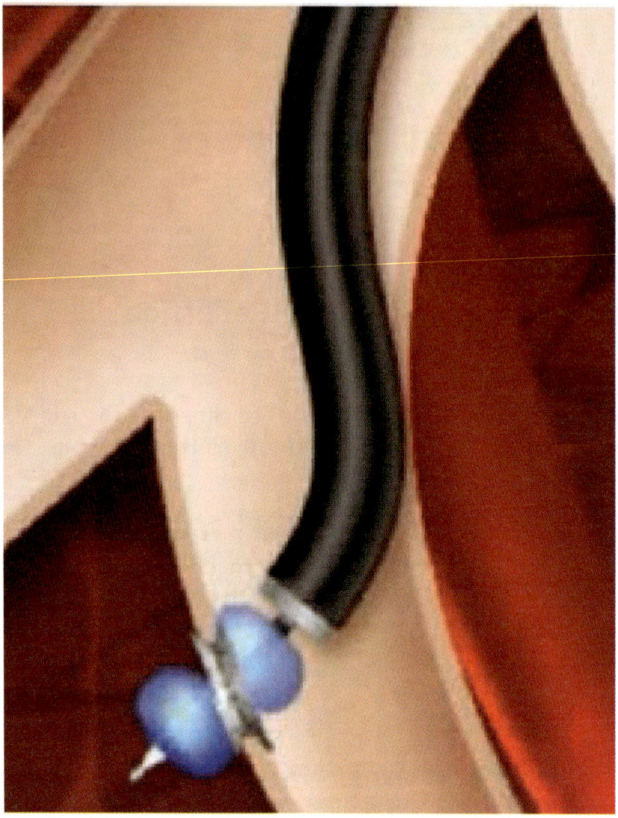

Figure 5.1 Airway bypass.

5.2 Airway Scaffold

Another similar proposal involves the bronchoscopic insertion of a novel self-expanding nitinol airway stent or BREATHE scaffold® (Apreo Health, CA, USA) into medium-sized subsegmental airways. In a similar idea to the airway bypass method, the scaffold is intended to prevent expiratory airway collapse. Thus, it is hoped that the hyperinflated distal emphysematous lung will empty more freely with less airway resistance present (Figure 5.2).

And does it work?

Yes, in the first-in-human studies in Australia (BREATHE-1) and in Europe (BREATHE-2), up to three scaffolds were implanted per lung

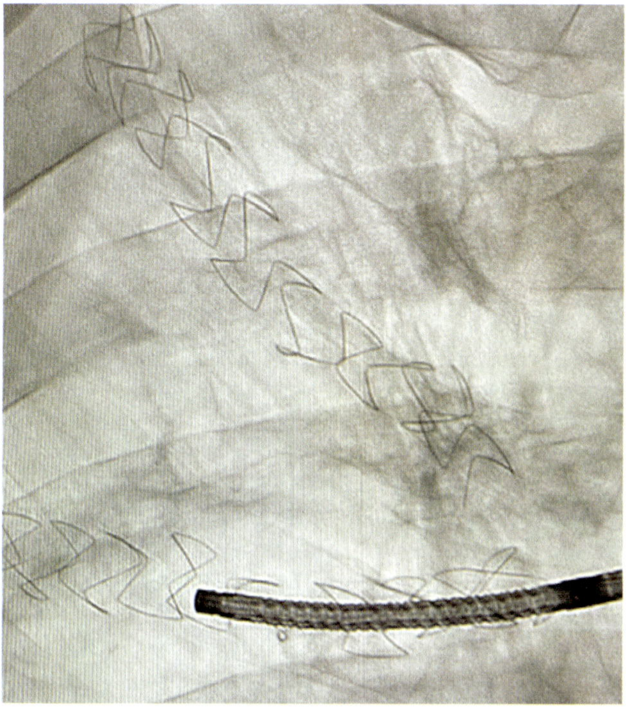

Figure 5.2 Airway scaffolds in situ. *Source*: Tane et al. (2025)/Oxford University Press.

in 50 patients with severe hyperinflation bilaterally and were found to achieve volume reduction by a significant drop in residual volume from baseline at 3 and 6 months [3].

What were the potential benefits compared to other methods?

The scaffolds were found to be effective even in patients with incomplete interlobar fissures (assumed to have collateral ventilation) and in those without at least a 15% difference between upper and lower lobes at −910 HU (assumed to be homogeneous). Unilateral homogeneous included one homogeneous and one heterogeneous lung. All groups showed improvement in the outcomes at 6 months, but those with at least one heterogeneous lung had a greater improvement. Fissure integrity did not have a significant impact on outcomes [4].

So, it may be an option for those potentially unsuitable for other endobronchial lung volume reduction (EBLVR) techniques due to incomplete fissures or homogenous emphysema.

Yes, but longer-term results and a randomized comparative trial are awaited.

Are there other proposed mechanisms for achieving EBLVR?

Yes, the next couple of methods are proposed to achieve volume reduction by direct action on the volume of the emphysematous lung parenchyma.

5.3 Vapour Ablation

Bronchoscopic thermal vapour ablation (BTVA) involves delivering heated water vapour to targeted emphysematous lung segments, inducing an inflammatory response that leads to lung volume reduction by shrinkage of the targeted segments due to the fibrotic reaction. BTVA could also increase elastic recoil by reducing the most compliant areas of the lung. Meanwhile, healthier segments should be preserved and allowed to expand after treatment to positively affect lung function, improve activity tolerance and preserve as much lung parenchyma as possible.

Ouch! Has this method been tested in a trial?

Yes, in using a staged bilateral approach in the STEP-UP study, 70% of patients achieved the minimal clinically important difference (MCID) in either forced expiratory volume in one second (FEV_1) or in the St George's Respiratory Questionnaire (SGRQ-C) at 6 months [5, 6].

Were there not safety concerns about "boiling" the lung?

The induced localized thermal inflammation appears to be responsible for acute exacerbation of COPD and pneumonia and is worse in the first 2–4 weeks and gradually resolves within 8–12 weeks. Radiographically, the targeted area will typically show infiltrates that are difficult to differentiate from pneumonia [7].

5.4 Endobronchial Coils

The RePneu® coil treatment (RePneu® coil system, PneumRx Inc./BTG, Santa Clara, CA, USA) is a bronchoscopic therapy for the treatment of patients with severe emphysema. The coil consists of a nickel-titanium alloy (nitinol), which exhibits a shape memory effect and is biologically inert (Figure 5.3).

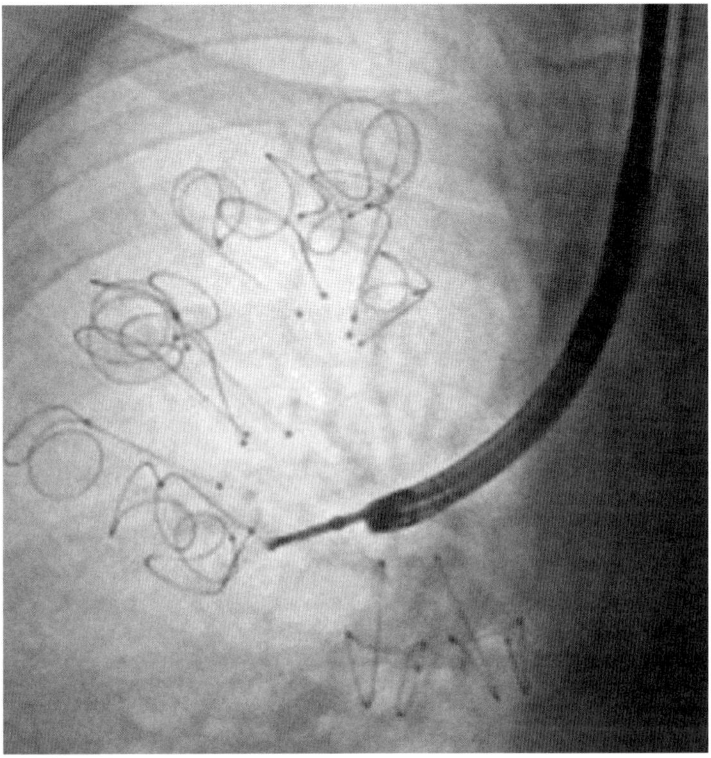

Figure 5.3 Endobronchial coils in situ. *Source*: Welling and Slebos (2018)/AME Publishing Company.

The proposed mechanism of action is by mechanical contraction, by release of the coil in the most hyperinflated emphysematous lung, achieving volume reduction and restoring elastic recoil. A similar improvement in chest wall mechanics to LVRS is asserted. There is also the claim that the coils act as a partial bronchial blocker, causing redistribution of airflow towards healthier parts of the lung [8].

Is there trial evidence for coils?

There have been three randomized trials comparing coils in a non-blinded fashion to best medical care: RESET [9], REVOLENS [10] and RENEW [11], with a 4th, ELEVATE [12], terminated prematurely for commercial reasons.

And was there a clinical benefit from this procedure?

Yes, modest but significant long-term improvements in quality of life and pulmonary function, but a shorter-term improvement in exercise

capacity. Importantly, half of the treated patients failed to reach at least one of the MCIDs (FEV_1, RV, SGRQ total score and 6MWD).

But I was aware of a worrying level of complications.

Serious adverse events, mainly major respiratory complications, occurred in 35% of coil patients and included pneumonia and pneumothorax. But mortality was not significantly elevated [13].

And what was the appropriate target population?

The benefits of coil treatment have been much greater in patients with severe hyperinflation and no significant comorbidity. However, the treatment is aimed at those with incomplete fissures and no significant heterogeneity, and on the other hand were associated with a higher likelihood of serious adverse events.

But these aren't the most common methods of obtaining EBLVR, are they?

No, the most widely used method is by causing volume reduction by lobar collapse, which is achieved by inserting one-way valves into the segmental bronchi. The resulting reduction in hyperinflation has favourable effects on chest wall mechanics and airflow obstruction.

5.5 Endobronchial Valves

We both know that the main factor used to determine which approach to LVR, and the major contraindication to endobronchial valves, is the presence of collateral ventilation (CV).

Yes, and let's summarize that this is the movement of air through channels that bypass the normal airways. The Channels of Martin are interbronchiolar pathways that connect adjacent bronchioles. They are larger than the pores of Kohn and the canals of Lambert, which are other pathways involved in collateral ventilation [14]. These are the channels most likely to result in interlobar collateral ventilation [15]. So, we assume that an incomplete interlobar fissure is associated with these communications, which prevent endobronchial blockage by valves from achieving lobar collapse. They open in emphysema as the airway resistance in normal airways is increased in the disease process above that of these channels.

I know that we can extrapolate from CT imaging and software analysis of fissure integrity the likelihood of CV, but there is a more direct method of assessment.

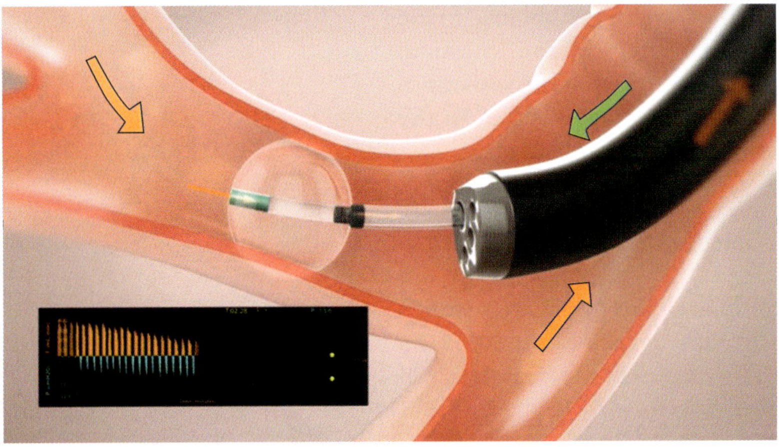

Figure 5.4 The Chartis® balloon occlusion catheter.

Yes, the Chartis® pulmonary assessment system (PulmonX, Redwood City, CA) (Figure 5.4) is an invasive, catheter-based measurement that is performed bronchoscopically, usually in the same setting before endobronchial valve placement. The catheter's balloon inflates and allows sealing of a pulmonary lobar bronchus with measurement of air pressure and flow from the sealed distal compartment. Persistence of flow after 5 minutes of balloon inflation suggests the presence of collateral ventilation to the sealed distal lobe.

Do we need to perform the Chartis assessment in all cases, or can we just rely on the CT software estimate?

It is suggested that when CT shows the fissure integrity to be <75%, it is likely that CV exists and that Chartis is not necessary. When the estimated fissure integrity is 75–90%, Chartis shows no CV in about one in three cases, so it is worth pursuing. However, when the fissure is more than 95% intact, Chartis can probably be omitted, particularly on the left [16].

How reliable is the Chartis method?

False-negative collateral ventilation assessment has been reported in a subset of patients, usually due to collapse of the bronchial wall distal to the inflated balloon. This is more likely in more severe emphysema, where the airways are more damaged, and they collapse prematurely when the positive pressure of ventilation is cut off. It has also been postulated that the presence of large collateral channels leads to reverse airflow, causing

air to escape from the target lobe to the adjacent lobe after balloon inflation. Again, this assumes that the resistance in normal airways exceeds that in the collateral channels.

5.5.1 Spiration Valve System

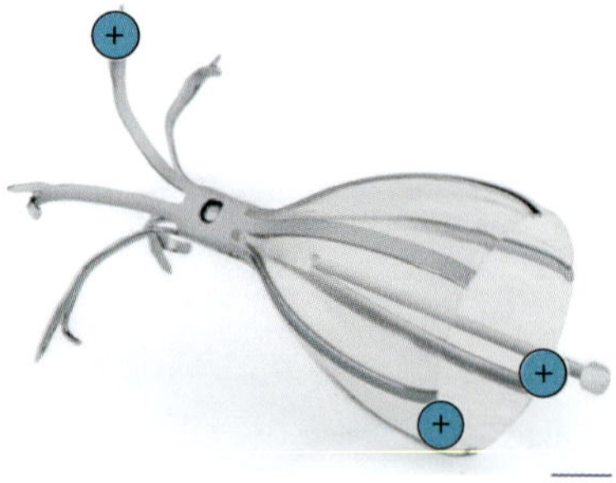

Figure 5.5 The Spiration umbrella intrabronchial valve.

The Spiration umbrella valve (Olympus America) was developed in 2008 and initially investigated in two randomized controlled trials: REACH [17] and EMPROVE [18] in nearly 400 patients (Figure 5.5).

In a subsequent meta-analysis of four randomized trials of the SVS, including 629 subjects, there were modest improvements in lung function, which were superior in those without collateral ventilation, but no significant improvement in exercise tolerance [19].

And similar respiratory complications to the other devices?

Yes. The serious adverse event rate was 33%, predominantly acute exacerbations of COPD. The incidence of pneumothoraxes requiring drainage was 26.5%.

Importantly, a valve dislocation rate of 24% was observed, but only in the lower lobes.

5.5.2 Zephyr Duckbill Valve

The Zephyr valve® (Pulmonx Inc., Redwood City, CA, USA) opens in expiration and closes in inspiration, allowing deflation of the target lobe. It is available in two sizes of valve in two lengths, which are tailored to the diameter of the segmental bronchus and depth of the segmental orifice (Figure 5.6).

What evidence is there for the efficacy of the Zephyr valve?

The Zephyr valve was initially developed and investigated by the VENT trial in 2007 in the United States [20] and Europe [21], but only modest and clinically not important benefits were achieved.

So, what made the difference to subsequent results?

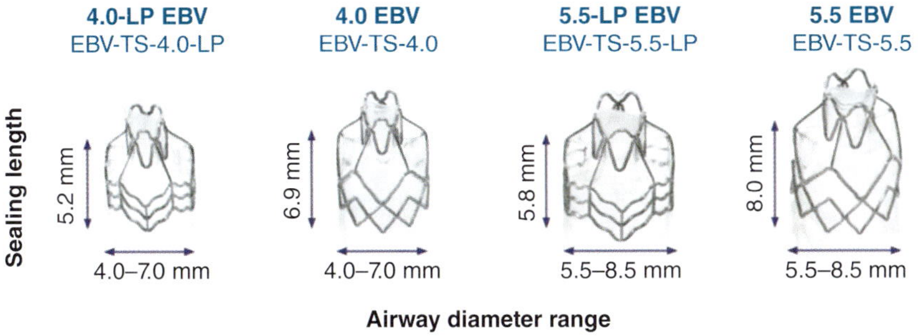

Figure 5.6 The Zephyr duckbill endobronchial valve.

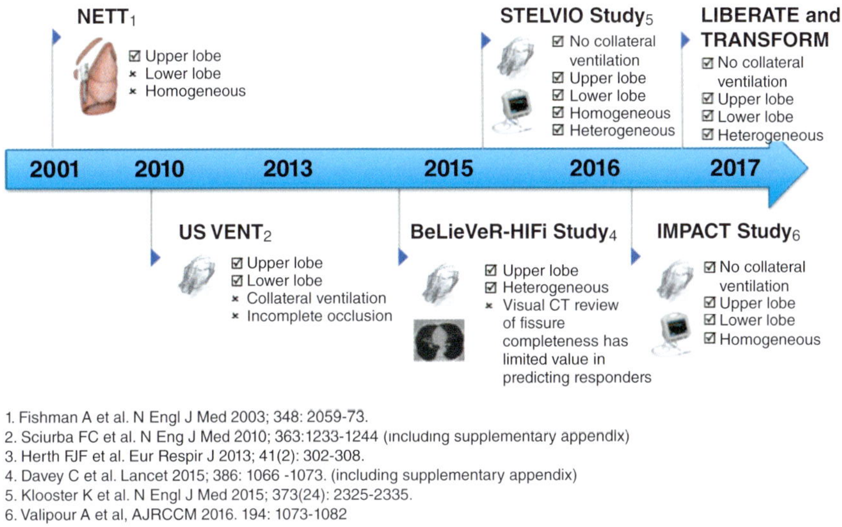

Figure 5.7 The timeline of the trial evidence for Zephyr valve.

In VENT, the outcomes were related to achieving the goal of lobar collapse and the importance of fissure integrity as seen on CT thorax. But in five subsequent trials (Figure 5.7) of nearly 500 patients, important lessons were learned.

In STELVIO [22] and BeLieVeR-HIFi [23], the importance of the Chartis assessment of collateral ventilation (CV) was confirmed, and in the latter trial, there was a significant risk shown from post EBLVR pneumothorax with mortality [24]. In IMPACT, the valves were shown to be of therapeutic benefit in those without standard heterogeneity and clear

target lobes, providing CV was not present [25]. Then, TRANSFORM [26] and LIBERATE [27] confirmed that the Zephyr valve gave significant and clinically relevant improvements in lung function, exercise capacity, physical activity, dyspnoea severity, and quality of life, and was reproducible in many centres.

But there are still some areas of debate around the use of the Zephyr valve.

5.6 Controversies

Is there any benefit from preoperative pulmonary rehabilitation (PR) before EBLVR?

One can understand why, in the absence of needing to recover after surgical incisions and chest drains, with earlier mobilization, one may think that it may not be essential. And one study suggests that the combination of PR before EBLVR did not result in additional improvement when compared to EBLVR alone [28]. However, the starting condition of the patient is probably the most important indication for the need for PR, and an individualized approach is suggested.

Is previous talc pleurodesis a contraindication to EBLVR using valves?

Two retrospective studies of patients treated in EBLVR trials have found an association between suspected pleural adhesions visible on CT with post EBLVR spontaneous pneumothorax (post EBLVR-SP) [29, 30]. This has then led to the suggestion in an expert consensus statement that valve placement is avoided in the presence of prior pleurodesis [31].

That doesn't make sense, surely prior talc pleurodesis (presumably for a previous spontaneous pneumothorax) would reduce the subsequent risk of post EBLVR-SP?

I agree, but there appears to be a theory that the target lobe will not collapse if it is held adherent to the apex of the chest.

Again, that does not make sense since the lobe will collapse if there is no ventilation to it, and the result of successful lung volume reduction is that the diaphragm ascends to regain its normal contour rather than the lung moving down away from the apex.

Well said.

Is the Chartis balloon occlusion catheter needed in all cases to exclude collateral ventilation? (Figure 5.4)

Well, it has been suggested that a fissure completion score in excess of 95% on the StratX software CT analysis of the left major fissure has a positive predictive value of 91% for the absence of CV, and therefore, Chartis can be omitted on the left. A multicentre observational study involving 240 EBLVR patients with pre-procedure quantitative CT analysis and a balloon occlusion physiological assessment noted increasing probability of collateral ventilation absence as fissure integrity scores increased and identified a left-sided minimal fissure score of 80% and a right-sided minimal score of 90%, below which all assessed fissures demonstrated collateral ventilation. Left major fissure scores exceeding 95% were associated with collateral ventilation in fewer than 10% [32].

But that runs the risk of nearly 1 in 10 patients in whom one places a valve, having CV and a likelihood of non-response.

Exactly, I can only think that there is an attraction in timesaving from omitting the Chartis procedure, which is probably more relevant when the patient is only sedated and may begin to cough or move. I also think that accepting anything other than complete occlusion and cessation of flow on the Chartis assessment should not be accepted as an indication to insert the valves.

Is there any benefit from using conscious sedation (CS) rather than general anaesthesia (GA) EBLVR?

Relevant to the above discussion, no benefit was found in using spontaneous ventilation rather than general anaesthesia [33]. The Chartis measurement under CS took significantly longer and required more measurements than under GA, without a difference in treatment outcome. It is worth noting that in the spontaneously ventilating patient, in order to save time, a flow volume trend of <6 ml/min in the last 20 seconds (VT20) can be used rather than waiting for the flow to diminish fully [34, 35].

5.7 Conclusions

What are the pros and cons of each of the endobronchial methods of lung volume reduction?

BTVA remains experimental, and concerns remain over short-term morbidity. Compared with valve treatment, the gradual effect of BTVA may result in a lower incidence of pneumothorax, and the absence of foreign body implants aids sputum clearance. But concerns remain over the initial tissue reaction to thermal damage with pneumonitis, exacerbation of COPD and loss of function. The proponents would say that the effects are gradual and, therefore, potentially make it safer than other minimally invasive modalities.

Airway bypass by creating new intrabronchial channels has largely been abandoned due to granulation tissue developing around stents and the subsequent difficulty in removing them to prevent infectious complications.

Airway scaffolds rely on the assumption that keeping existing large to medium-sized airways patent with a stent-like device will encourage deflation by preventing expiratory airway collapse. A criticism would be that the compliant, inelastic peripheral lung parenchyma is unlikely to deflate passively through the opened airways. It is conceivable that inspiratory flow may be facilitated by the stented airways, thus paradoxically increasing hyperinflation. There are also concerns, as for airway bypass, regarding infectious complications from blocked stents and the difficulties in removing them. Their presence also negates the possibility of surgical LVRS salvage in non-response unless lobectomy is contemplated.

Endobronchial coils result in relatively low levels of volume reduction and may be limited in application to the best candidates with the most hyperinflation and most heterogeneous disease distribution. Although there are promotions for those who are CV positive. There remains no clear indication regarding the number and distribution of the coils or any 'dose response'. As with the stents, their removal is unlikely, thus precluding further intervention, i.e. salvage LVRS. It is also worth noting that to achieve satisfactory results and minimize adverse events requires a high level of technical competency and equipment.

The attraction of all of these methods in comparison to endobronchial valves is the apparent low risk of treatment-related pneumothorax and application even in the presence of collateral ventilation. However, the evidence of efficacy is less robust than for endobronchial valves. They also have their own specific risk factors.

But which of the two types of valves is superior?

There has been no head-to-head trial comparing both valve systems, and no clear benefit of one over the other in terms of physiological outcome in the absence of CV. However, only the Zephyr valve has proven efficacy in patients with homogeneous emphysema, and it is the only FDA-approved valve for this group [36]. Furthermore, the Umbrella valve has been associated with a similar rate of pneumothorax as the Zephyr valve but a higher rate of dislocation and displacement.

So, the only validated technique for EBLVR is the use of one-way endobronchial valves, and the remainder remain in the clinical trial setting.

Indeed, but the Achilles Heel of the valves is collateral ventilation, and the future research is to be directed at either addressing techniques to close these collateral interlobar channels of ventilation or to perfect an endobronchial device that can function in their presence.

References

1 Choong CK, Macklem PT, Pierce JA, Das N, Lutey BA, Martinez CO, et al. Airway bypass improves the mechanical properties of explanted emphysematous lungs. Am J Respir Crit Care Med. 2008 Nov 1;178(9):902–905.
2 Shah PL, Slebos DJ, Cardoso PF, Cetti E, Voelker K, Levine B, et al. Bronchoscopic lung-volume reduction with Exhale airway stents for emphysema (EASE trial): randomised, sham-controlled, multicentre trial. Lancet. 2011 Sep 10;378(9795): 997–1005.
3 Tana A, Valipour A, Ing A, Steinfort DP, Orton CM, Klooster K, et al. Airway Scaffolds for Emphysema-related Hyperinflation: Six-Month Results from the BREATHE Trial. Am J Respir Crit Care Med. 2025 Jul;211(7):1175–1184.
4 Tana A, Valipour A, Ing A, Steinfort DP, Orton CM, Garner JL, et al. P210 The impact of heterogeneity and fissure integrity on the treatment response of Airway Scaffolds for emphysema-related hyperinflation. Thorax. 2025;80(Suppl 2): A278.1-A278.
5 Herth FJ, Valipour A, Shah PL, Eberhardt R, Grah C, Egan J, et al. Segmental volume reduction using thermal vapour ablation in patients with severe emphysema: 6-month results of the multicentre, parallel-group, open-label, randomised controlled STEP-UP trial. Lancet Respir Med. 2016;4:185–193.
6 Gompelmann D, Eberhardt R, Schuhmann M, Valipour A, Shah PL, Herth FJ, et al. Lung volume reduction with vapor ablation in the presence of incomplete fissures: 12-month results from the step-up randomized controlled study. Respiration. 2016;92:397–403.
7 Zhi L, Liao L, Wu Z, Wang T, Ye Y, Li H, et al. Impact of bronchoscopic thermal vapor ablation on lung volume reduction in patients with emphysema: a meta-analysis. BMC Pulm Med. 2023 Oct 26;23(1):405.
8 Welling JBA, Slebos DJ. Lung volume reduction with endobronchial coils for patients with emphysema. J Thorac Dis. 2018 Aug;10(Suppl 23):S2797–S2805.
9 Shah PL, Zoumot Z, Singh S, Bicknell SR, Ross ET, Quiring J, et al. Endobronchial coils for the treatment of severe emphysema with hyperinflation (RESET): a randomised controlled trial. Lancet Respir Med. 2013 May;1(3):233–240.

10 Deslée G, Mal H, Dutau H, Bourdin A, Vergnon JM, Pison C, et al. Lung volume reduction coil treatment vs usual care in patients with severe emphysema: the revolens randomized clinical trial. JAMA. 2016 Jan 12;315(2):175–184.

11 Sciurba FC, Criner GJ, Strange C, Shah PL, Michaud G, Connolly TA, et al. Effect of endobronchial coils vs usual care on exercise tolerance in patients with severe emphysema: the renew randomized clinical trial. JAMA. 2016 May 24–31; 315(20):2178–2189.

12 Klooster K, Valipour A, Marquette CH, Boutros J, Mal H, Marceau A, et al. Endobronchial coil system versus standard-of-care medical management in the treatment of subjects with severe emphysema. Respiration. 2021;100(8):804–810.

13 Slebos DJ, Hartman JE, Klooster K, Blaas S, Deslee G, Gesierich W, et al. Bronchoscopic coil treatment for patients with severe emphysema: a meta-analysis. Respiration. 2015;90(2):136–145.

14 Terry PB, Traystman RJ, Newball HH, Batra G, Menkes HA. Collateral ventilation in man. N Engl J Med. 1978 Jan 5;298(1):10–15.

15 Koster TD, Slebos DJ. The fissure: interlobar collateral ventilation and implications for endoscopic therapy in emphysema. Int J Chron Obstruct Pulmon Dis. 2016 Apr 13;11:765–773.

16 Fiorelli A, Santini M, Shah P. When can computed tomography-fissure analysis replace Chartis collateral ventilation assessment in the prediction of patients with emphysema who might benefit from endobronchial valve therapy? Interact Cardiovasc Thorac Surg. 2018 Feb 1;26(2):313–318.

17 Li S, Wang G, Wang C, Gao X, Jin F, Yang H, et al. The reach trial: a randomized controlled trial assessing the safety and effectiveness of the spiration® valve system in the treatment of severe emphysema. Respiration. 2019;97(5):416–427.

18 Hogarth DK, Delage A, Zgoda MA, Nsiah-Dosu S, Himes D, Reed MF. Efficacy and safety of the spiration valve system™ for the treatment of severe emphysema in patients with Alpha-1 antitrypsin deficiency (EMPROVE). Respir Med. 2024 Apr; 224:107565.

19 Majid A, Labarca G, Uribe JP, Kheir F, Pacheco C, Folch E, et al. Efficacy of the spiration valve system in patients with severe heterogeneous emphysema: a systematic review and meta-analysis. Respiration. 2020;99(1):62–72.

20 Sciurba FC, Ernst A, Herth FJ, Strange C, Criner GJ, Marquette CH, et al. A randomized study of endobronchial valves for advanced emphysema. N Engl J Med. 2010 Sep 23;363(13):1233–1244.

21 Herth FJ, Noppen M, Valipour A, Leroy S, Vergnon JM, Ficker JH, et al. Efficacy predictors of lung volume reduction with Zephyr valves in a European cohort. Eur Respir J. 2012 Jun;39(6):1334–1342.

22 Klooster K, Ten Hacken NH, Hartman JE, Kerstjens HA, van Rikxoort EM, Slebos DJ. Endobronchial valves for emphysema without interlobar collateral ventilation. N Engl J Med. 2015;373:2325–2335.

23 Davey C, Zoumot Z, Jordan S, McNulty WH, Carr DH, Hind MD, et al. Bronchoscopic lung volume reduction with endobronchial valves for patients with heterogeneous emphysema and intact interlobar fissures (the BeLieVeR-HIFi study): a randomised controlled trial. Lancet. 2015;386(9998):1066–1073.

24 Shrager JB. Endobronchial valves in a highly parsed emphysema population. Lancet. 2015;386(9998):1022–1023.

25 Eberhardt R, Slebos DJ, Herth FJF, Darwiche K, Wagner M, Ficker JH, et al. Endobronchial valve (zephyr) treatment in homogeneous emphysema: one-year results from the impact randomized clinical trial. Respiration. 2021;100(12):1174–1185.

26 Kemp SV, Slebos DJ, Kirk A, Kornaszewska M, Carron K, Ek L, et al. A multicenter randomized controlled trial of zephyr endobronchial valve treatment in heterogeneous emphysema (TRANSFORM). Am J Respir Crit Care Med. 2017 Dec 15;196(12):1535–1543.

27 Criner GJ, Sue R, Wright S, Dransfield M, Rivas-Perez H, Wiese T, et al. A multicenter randomized controlled trial of zephyr endobronchial valve treatment in heterogeneous emphysema (LIBERATE). Am J Respir Crit Care Med. 2018 Nov 1;198(9):1151–1164.

28 Posthuma R, van der Molen MC, Vaes AW, Hartman JE, Spruit MA, Slebos DJ, et al. The impact of bronchoscopic lung volume reduction with endobronchial valves with or without pulmonary rehabilitation on symptoms of fatigue, anxiety and depression: a multicentre randomised controlled trial. ERJ Open Res. 2025 Aug 11;11(4):00892–2024.

29 van Geffen WH, Klooster K, Hartman JE, Ten Hacken NHT, Kerstjens HAM, Wolf RFE, et al. Pleural adhesion assessment as a predictor for pneumothorax after endobronchial valve treatment. Respiration. 2017;94(2):224–231.

30 Gompelmann D, Lim HJ, Eberhardt R, Gerovasili V, Herth FJ, Heussel CP, et al. Predictors of pneumothorax following endoscopic valve therapy in patients with severe emphysema. Int J Chron Obstruct Pulmon Dis. 2016 Aug 1;11:1767–1773.

31 Wahidi MM, Lentz RJ, Criner GJ, Gompelmann D, Ing AJ, Kapp CM, et al. Bronchoscopic lung volume reduction with endobronchial valves: a consensus statement on the practical aspects of patient selection and periprocedural management. Respiration. 2025 Sep 15:1–33.

32 Klooster K, Koster TD, Ruwwe-Glösenkamp C, Theilig D, Doellinger F, Saccomanno J, et al. An integrative approach of the fissure completeness score and chartis assessment in endobronchial valve treatment for emphysema. Int J Chron Obstruct Pulmon Dis. 2020 Jun 9;15:1325–1334.

33 Welling JBA, Hartman JE, Ten Hacken NHT, Franz I, Charbonnier JP, van Rikxoort EM, et al. Chartis measurement of collateral ventilation: conscious sedation versus general anesthesia – a retrospective comparison. Respiration. 2018;96(5):480–487.

34 Koster TD, Klooster K, McNamara H, Shargill NS, Radhakrishnan S, Olivera R, et al. An adjusted and time-saving method to measure collateral ventilation with Chartis. ERJ Open Res. 2021 Jul 26;7(3):00191–2021.

35 Saccomanno J, Sgarbossa T, Pappe E, Kilic L, Biglari S, Shargill NS, et al. VT20 method for Chartis assessment of collateral ventilation with flexible bronchoscopy under procedural sedation. ERJ Open Res. 2024 Jul 8;10(4): 00945–2023.

36 Nada KM, Nishi S. Endoscopic lung volume reduction: review of the EMPROVE and LIBERATE trials. Mayo Clin Proc Innov Qual Outcomes. 2020 Dec 11;5(1): 177–186.

6

Which Technique and Why?

6.1 Collateral Ventilation

Surgeon: So, in the choice of procedure, we can agree that lung volume reduction surgery (LVRS) is applicable to all who fulfil the physiological and radiological selection criteria, whereas endobronchial lung volume reduction (EBLVR) is limited by the presence of collateral ventilation.

Pulmonologist: Well, I agree that CV has traditionally been a contraindication to EBLVR, but as we will discuss later, there are developing techniques designed to combat CV by endobronchial methods. But fundamentally, EBLVR is more attractive to the patient. They are fearful of an operation, a prolonged stay in hospital and long-term pain.

6.2 Comparative Risk/Cost of the Procedures

Let me address the concern that LVRS is of a higher risk than EBLVR. Where is the evidence for that assumption?

The 90-day mortality rate in the National Emphysema Treatment Trial (NETT) was 7.9% [1], whereas in the LIBERATE trial of endobronchial valves, the in-hospital mortality was only 3% [2].

The data in the NETT is not comparable with the modern practice of LVRS. As discussed in Chapter 4, median sternotomy and bilateral surgery have now been superseded by minimally invasive unilateral LVRS with a significant reduction in risk. Indeed, a recent retrospective analysis of the Medicare/Medicaid database found that EBV procedures have higher risk-adjusted mortality and procedure-related morbidity despite fewer comorbidities than patients undergoing LVRS [3].

Ok, I accept that newer surgical management techniques may have reduced the risk, together with better selection. But the patients still have to stay in the hospital longer.

The average length of stay is coming down for LVRS and is around 7 days, but even after EBLVR using valves, they need to stay for 3 days because of the risk of pneumothorax (to be discussed in Chapter 7). If that does occur, then the hospital stay can be longer than for LVRS [4].

But the majority will have a shorter hospital episode, which will also be more attractive to the hospital authorities. Also, the risk of pneumothorax may be predicted, and therefore avoided, or the clinician may insert a prophylactic drain to allow same-day discharge (see Chapter 7).

However, there is an increased cost of consumables associated with the devices used for EBLVR. This offsets any savings in bed days as readmission is more common after EBLVR [4] for valve-related complications (see Chapter 7). In fact, LVRS by VATS is probably the most cost-effective method of LVR ahead of RATS or EBLVR. Irrespective of the initial outlay on the technology, the running costs for VATS are lower than RATS [5].

6.3 Physiological Outcomes

Furthermore, LVRS is a more physiologically justifiable technique than EBLVR since it follows the original mantra of removing the most functionless lung. Valves aim for entire lobar collapse, but LVRS retains the more functional part of the lobe.

However, in the only randomized trial of its kind, The CELEB trial: Comparative Effectiveness of Lung volume reduction surgery for Emphysema and Bronchoscopic lung volume reduction with valve placement in UK, there was no difference in the improvement in the i-BODE nor in its individual components between LVRS and EBLVR. I do concede that there was a similar mortality risk between each treatment arm [6].

That is true, but the criticisms of the CELEB trial include the fact that it was only powered to show non-inferiority for EBLVR due to the relatively small numbers of participants. It should also be noted that the only significant difference in the outcomes between LVRS and EBLVR was in the CAT score measurement of quality of life. This was higher at 6 and 12 months in the LVRS group, possibly because of the non-response rate in the EBLVR arm and their need for revision?

Are there any other physiological considerations that may influence the decision between EBLVR and LVRS?

A relatively unexplored variable is how well perfused does the target lobe have to be to for it to be a contraindication to lobar EBLVR?

Yes, there must be a risk of increasing the ventilation: perfusion mismatch if a well-perfused lobe is occluded and collapsed by EBLVR. But I am not aware of any critical cut-off value for the percentage perfusion of the target lobe above which EBLVR should not be attempted. I suppose that the benefit of endobronchial valves is that they can be removed post-primary procedure if oxygen desaturation, particularly on exercise, becomes a problem.

That is true and I am aware of the IMPACT study when valves were placed into relatively well-perfused lobes with less than 20% difference in inter-lobar heterogeneity with satisfactory results [7].

Would you always insist on a preoperative perfusion scan in the selection between methods?

Yes, I would and this opinion is not held by a consensus of expert pulmonologists who view the perfusion scan as optional [8]. I prefer the single-photon emission computed tomography (SPECT) scans, which gives an anatomical appreciation of the lobar perfusion and may identity intralobar heterogeneity with well-perfused parts of a lobe but potential peripheral targets. This is an indication for targeted LVRS, not hopeful EBLVR.

So, where the patient may be suitable for both LVRS and EBLVR, how would you summarize your selection process?

I would always prioritize the functional effects of the procedure over any perceived benefits from the less invasive procedure. Case Study 1 illustrates the dilemma.

And to reopen the unilateral vs bilateral LVR debate. How would you manage bilateral targets? Case Study 2 is an example of this discussion.

6.4 Future Trials

I guess that you surgeons were a little disappointed with the results of the CELEB trial, so I understand that there is a new proposal for a further randomized comparison.

Yes, the SINCERE (Surgical Compared to Bronchoscopic Lung Volume Reduction in Patients with Severe Emphysema) trial (NCT04537182) is a multicentre European trial which will compare bilateral lung volume reduction surgery (LVRS) with bronchoscopic lung volume reduction (BLVR) using endobronchial valves in terms of efficacy and patient safety.

That doesn't sound sensible to compare bilateral with unilateral LVR? A little bias from the surgeons, perhaps.

I agree. I think the choice may have been influenced by the existing surgical protocols in the participating units. Nevertheless, it will make interpretation and application of the results more difficult. I guess you pulmonologists will make the most of it.

We will undoubtedly, but it does present other potential problems. The outcome data will only be collected for up to 12 months.

Yes, I foresee a criticism because any potential decline after bilateral LVR or the potential for further treatment may not be fully appreciated. I note also that bronchoscopic Chartis® measurement of collateral ventilation will not be mandated if fissure completeness according to StratX® exceeds 95%. Again, that is potentially favouring surgery?

This may risk non-responders in the EBLVR group and bias the results even further. What about targets? Will only heterogeneous emphysema be included?

No, all morphology on CT and perfusion scan, if performed. Which I suppose will favour LVRS again, since evidence of intralobar heterogeneity but lack of interlobar heterogeneity may push one towards recommending LVRS rather than EBLVR.

Not necessarily. The IMPACT trial assessed the effectiveness of the Zephyr valve in a diagnosis of homogeneous emphysema based on a difference in the emphysema destruction scores (heterogeneity index using −910 HU cutoff) between target and adjacent lobes of between target and adjacent lobes of between target and adjacent lobes of <15%, and an absolute difference in perfusion (using perfusion scintigraphy) between right and left lungs of ≤20%. Clinically meaningful benefits were found at 12 months follow-up [7].

But collateral ventilation remains the Achilles heel of EBLVR.

At present, but in the future, there will be alternative methods of LVR that are not dependent on the lack of collateral ventilation. These are other endobronchial techniques under evaluation, including a new version of the self-expanding endobronchial coil and an airway scaffold-like stent, which have the potential advantages over valves (see Chapter 5, where we have discussed their relative merits).

But the valves are the preferred device for EBLVR, so do you have any method of increasing their application?

Well, we pulmonologists may have a non-invasive method to combat collateral ventilation. Initial studies suggest that it may be possible to block the collateral channels of Martin with bronchoscopic application of a foam containing a tissue glue-like material, Aeriseal. Although this process may require several applications. It is currently under evaluation in the CONVERT II trial (NCT06035120).

We surgeons may also have a solution to the problem of collateral ventilation.

I guess that you will need to do LVRS in these patients?

That is certainly what I used to do, but without removing the in-dwelling valves. Then it occurred to me: why not just divide the interlobar fissure, removing any possible channels for CV, and facilitating the placement of valves?

6.5 Fissure Division

Why would you consider that instead of the established surgical technique?

Potentially just dividing the incomplete fissure would lead to reduced air leak compared to conventional LVRS. Not only would it involve fewer staple lines but would also divide only collateral channels rather than functioning lung parenchyma with larger airways. Also, any chance of an induced air leak in the target lobe distal to the staple lines would be eliminated if target lobe collapse was achieved with the valves.

But you would still be at risk of valve-related complications, including postprocedural pneumothorax from the non-target lobe.

That's true, but the patient would already wake up with an indwelling chest drain, and during the fissure division, any likely culprit bullae in the non-target lobe can be resected, further reducing the risk of postoperative air leak.

That sounds sensible. But is there not a risk from dissecting in the fissure in the emphysematous lung?

Data is limited at present, but I would point out that thoracic surgeons have to divide the interlobar fissure routinely in lung cancer operations. The dissection is facilitated by robotic-assisted thoracic surgery (RATS). The technique of fissure division has been shown to be feasible and effective in the animal model [9] and in a small human series [10]. One feasibility study has been completed in Australia [10] where VATS fissure division was completed first and if successful, the patients went onto have endobronchial valves inserted at a second procedure 2 weeks later [11].

That sounds quite a big undertaking for the patients.

I suggest that the endobronchial valves should be inserted first under the same general anaesthetic, then proceed with minimally invasive surgery and fissure division. The benefit of this order is that the target lobe collapse can be confirmed in vivo by reinflating the lung with the camera in the chest. Case study 3 illustrates this procedure.

That again makes sense, but I would want to see the potential benefits in a feasibility study before applying it more widely. Particularly to treatment naïve, CV-positive patients. And in these, should you divide the fissure first before inserting the valves?

Yes, and there is at least one prospective trial ongoing in the United States [12] with more planned in the United Kingdom and France.

I hope these are successful, as there seem to be many potential benefits from this "hybrid" approach.

There are many, including: reducing the postoperative air leak and hospital stay after LVRS; reducing the possibility of non-response after EBLVR, and increasing collaboration between surgeons and pulmonologists.

Well said...

6.6 CASE STUDY 1: The Choice Between EBLVR and LVRS

In this 67-year-old patient, the physiological selection criteria are met: FEV_1 805 ml (32% predicted), RV 205% predicted, loss of diffusion capacity (DLCO) 29% predicted. He has no echocardiographic evidence of ventricular dysfunction and no respiratory failure with pO_2 8.1 kPa, pCO_2 6.4 kPa. His body mass index (BMI) is 21.

SUMMARY

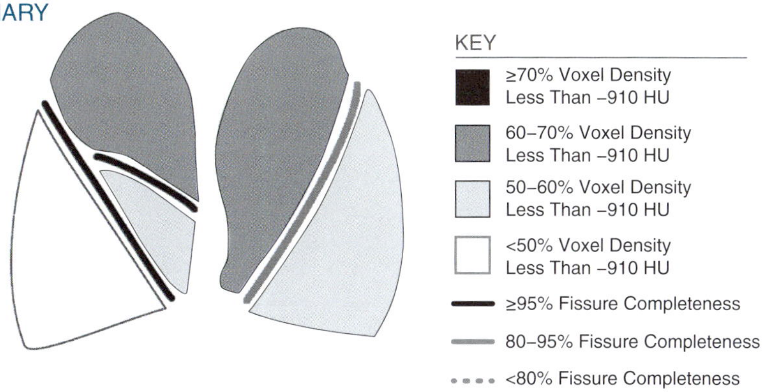

RESULTS

	RIGHT LUNG				LEFT LUNG	
	RUL	RUL + RML	RML	RLL	LUL	LLL
% Fissure Completeness	98.8	99.7	99.0	99.7	83.1	83.1
% Voxel Density Less Than −910 HU	65	64	54	27	64	50
% Voxel Density Less Than −950 HU	37	34	16	6	35	24
Inspiratory Volume (ml)	1215	1393	178	1218	978	1264

I note several facts from his StratX software report: there appear to be good bilateral upper lobe targets with high emphysema scores (>30% −950 HU) and interlobar heterogeneity (more marked on the right) on HRCT; fissure integrity is high on the major and minor right fissures, but the left fissure is incomplete. The largest lobe is the left lower, but the right upper is larger than the left upper.

What would you offer the patient?

Well, assuming he is of acceptable risk (I calculate a Glenfield score of only 1), the fissure integrity is greater on the RIGHT, so I would suggest RIGHT upper lobe EBLVR, but it would depend on a negative balloon catheter assessment of collateral ventilation.

Would you ask for a perfusion scan?

Yes, I would in this case, as there are multilobar potential targets on CT analysis, and the emphysema severity in the assumed target of the right upper lobe is not the most severe, i.e. only 37% <−950 HU.

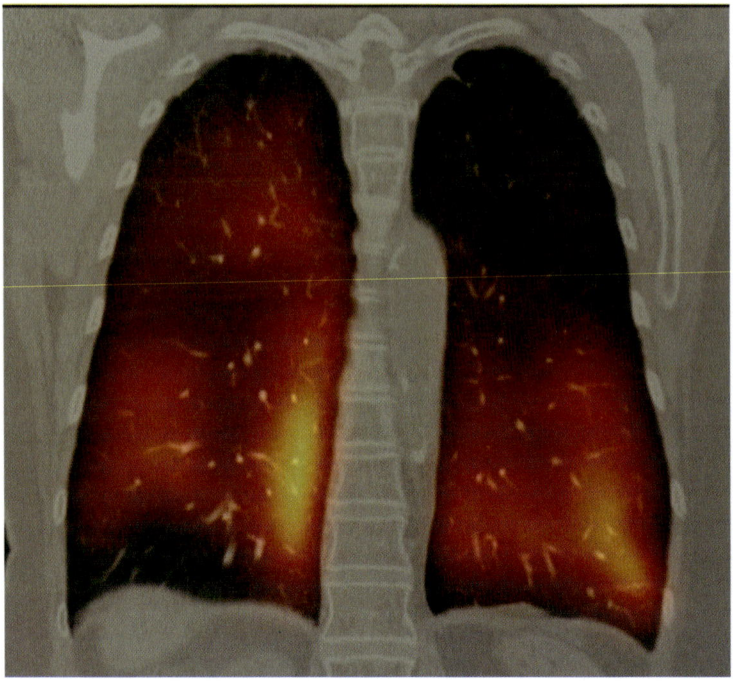

Well, we did obtain a perfusion scan. Does this help your decision?

The SPECT scan demonstrates a marked perfusion difference between the upper lobes, with the clearest target in the LEFT upper lobe.

Do you favour the less invasive technique on the RIGHT or the more physiological but subjectively more invasive operation on the LEFT?

I would offer the patient the alternatives of RIGHT EBLVR with a risk that the valves may need to be removed due to possible postoperative hypoxia secondary to intrapulmonary arteriovenous shunting from ventilation: perfusion or LEFT LVRS.

The patient opted for LEFT upper lobe LVRS and had a good outcome. The principle here is that the preservation of a functioning lung outweighs the perceived benefit of a less invasive procedure. Long-term benefit over short-term gain.

6.7 CASE STUDY 2: Bilateral Targets

This 74-year-old female patient was severely hyperinflated (RV 250% predicted), but with suitable lung function: FEV_1 790 ml (28% predicted) and DLCO 26% predicted. She had neither significant cardiac dysfunction nor any evidence of respiratory failure.

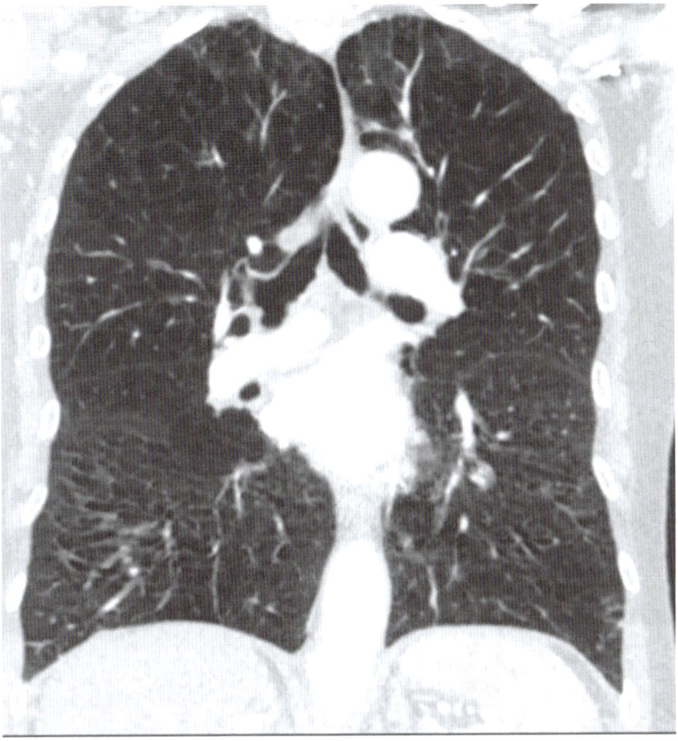

Her CT shows bilateral severe emphysema in both upper lobes with the suggestion of well-preserved fissure integrity.

SUMMARY

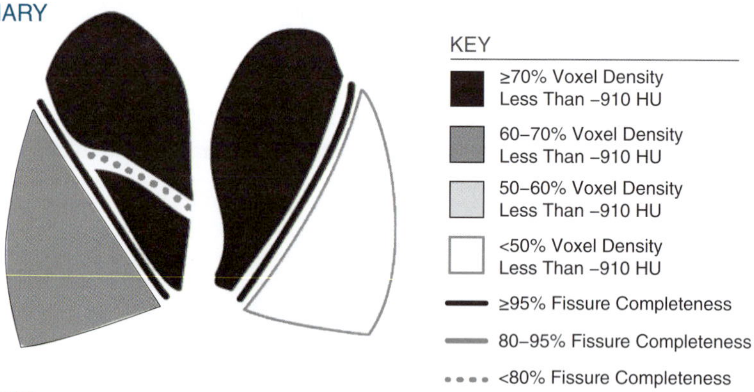

RESULTS

	RIGHT LUNG				LEFT LUNG	
	RUL	RUL + RML	RML	RLL	LUL	LLL
% Fissure Completeness	73.8	96.1	76.6	96.1	95.3	95.3
% Voxel Density Less Than –910 HU	81	80	77	61	73	49
% Voxel Density Less Than –950 HU	62	60	55	35	44	23
Inspiratory Volume (ml)	1517	2109	592	1846	1750	1434

Absolutely, confirmed on the StratX® software analysis. Severe upper lobe emphysema is probably worse on the RIGHT (62% <–950 HU) with good fissure integrity (>95%) on both major fissures. Are you ready to make a decision?

I am favouring RIGHT EBLVR, which will probably entail blocking both upper and middle lobes. While some may say a perfusion scan is optional, as there are bilateral targets, I would want a comparative perfusion score.

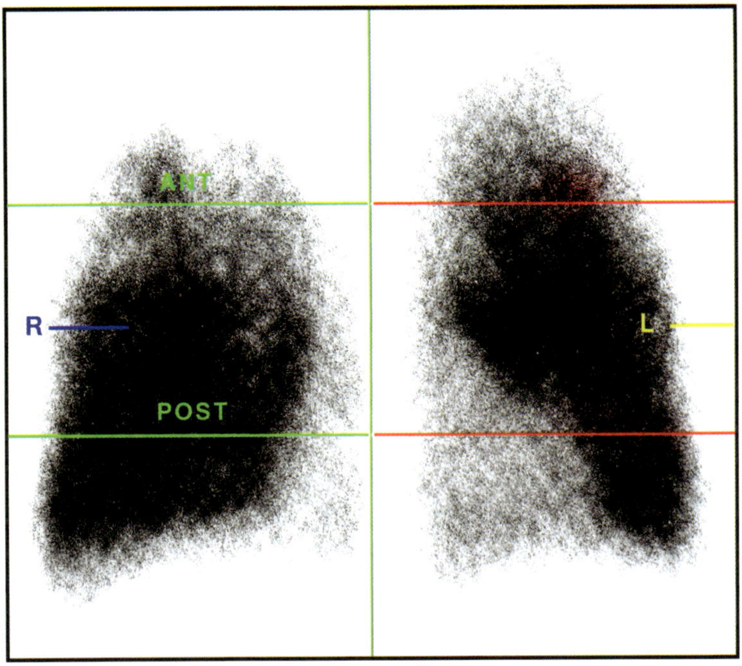

The planar lung perfusion scintigraphy identifies clear bilateral upper lobe targets with slightly more perfusion on the RIGHT.

Then the plan still holds for RIGHT EBLVR.

Would you check for collateral ventilation with a Chartis® assessment?

Yes, I note the Fissure Completion Score on the LEFT is just over 95%, but I would perform BILATERAL checks for CV.

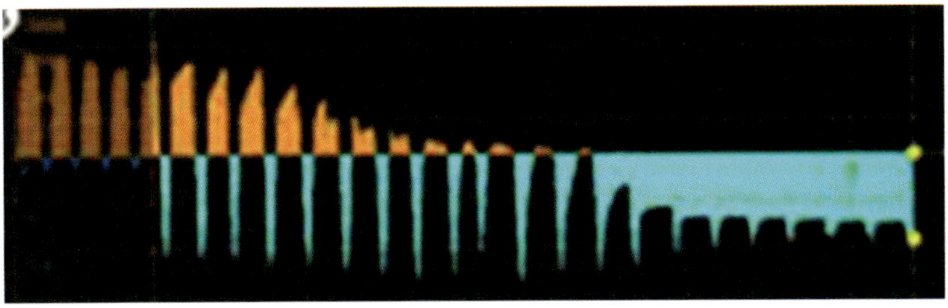

Under GA, the Chartis® catheter was inserted into the right LOWER lobe to measure CV across the major fissure. As the minor (horizontal) fissure was very incomplete, it was decided not to attempt just the right upper lobe EBLVR.

The trace shows no evidence of CV, so I would go ahead with valves in all upper five segments on the RIGHT.

Are you concerned about the disease severity in the non-target lung?

Yes, I am aware of the emphysema severity in the RIGHT lower lobe (35% <−950 HU) and the relatively large volume, which increase ethe risk of post EBLVR pneumothorax.

Any other concerns?

Well, the left upper lobe remains severely emphysematous, so there is a real risk of compensatory hyperinflation in that lobe, which may adversely affect the outcome.

I agree. I know of many surgeons who would advocate one-stage bilateral LVRS in this type of situation.

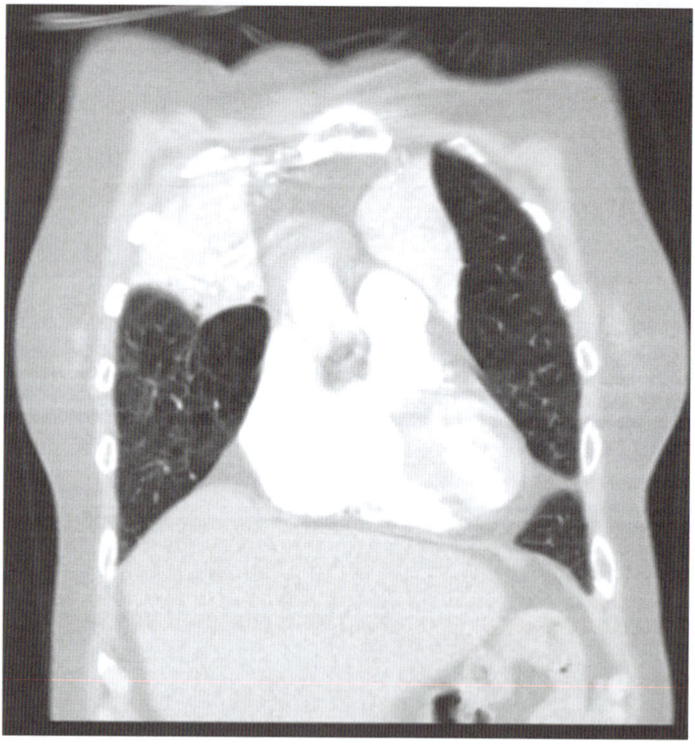

We actually planned sequential EBLVR with the RIGHT upper and middle lobes at the first operation. There were no postoperative complications. Successful collapse of the upper five right segments was achieved with five separate Zephyr valves with a good clinical outcome.

LEFT upper lobe EBLVR was successfully performed 3 months later, achieving bilateral upper lobe collapse as above.

6.8 CASE STUDY 3: A Higher Risk Case with a Treatment Dilemma

A 77-year-old female has become severely more breathless over the last 12 months, and her independent living is now threatened. She is very motivated to undergo treatment.

She fulfils the criteria for LVR but is in the moderate risk category (Glenfield score of 4): RV 260% predicted, FEV_1 550 ml (19% predicted), diffusion capacity(TLCO) 19% predicted, BMI 21 kg/m^2.

SUMMARY

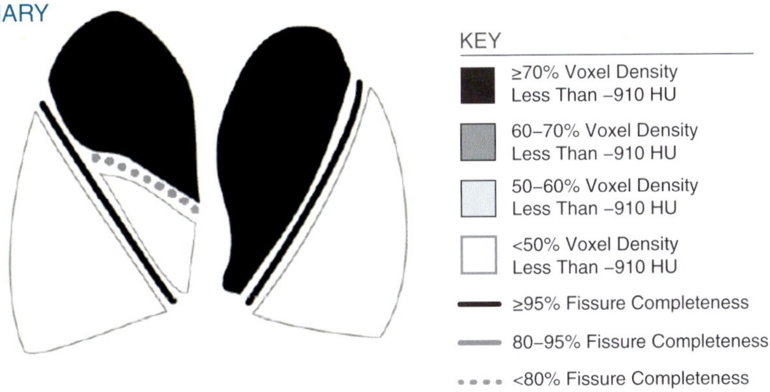

RESULTS

	RIGHT LUNG				LEFT LUNG	
	RUL	RUL + RML	RML	RLL	LUL	LLL
% Fissure Completeness	96.7	−1.0	−1.0	96.7	98.4	98.4
% Voxel Density Less Than −910 HU	77	−1	−1	20	72	17
% Voxel Density Less Than −950 HU	60	−1	−1	11	56	9
Inspiratory Volume (ml)	1699	−1	−1	1009	1449	807

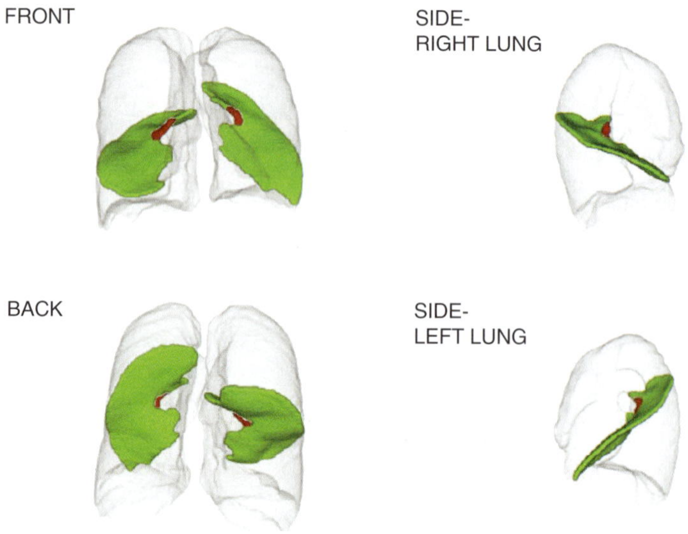

Her CT analysis demonstrates severe emphysema in both upper lobes with high interlobar heterogeneity. As the fissure integrity is high we can explain that there is a very good chance of EBLVR.

Her lung perfusion was 5% better in the LEFT UPPER LOBE compared to the right, so she was prepared for RIGHT UPPER and MIDDLE lobe EBLVR (as the minor fissure is incomplete).

She asked what we will do if the valves cannot be placed. She wanted a definitive one-stage procedure. LVRS was discussed, but she was aware of the increased risk due to her frailty and was keen to leave the hospital as soon as possible.

Under general anaesthesia, we carried out the Chartis® balloon catheter assessment of collateral ventilation across the right major fissure.

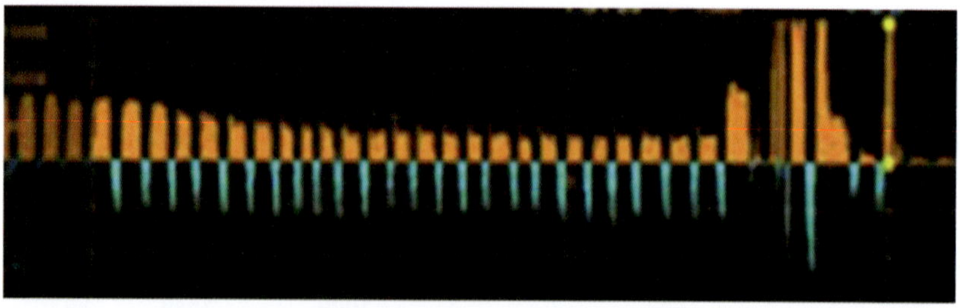

The trace above from the occlusion catheter assessment in the right lower lobe demonstrates persistent distal flow, indicating collateral ventilation between the right lower and upper/middle lobes. We could therefore consider the LEFT upper lobe EBLVR.

Unfortunately, the trace was similar on the LEFT suggesting collateral ventilation was also present on this side.

So, did you proceed?

Yes, preoperatively, we had offered the alternative of one-stage endobronchial valve placement with fissure division if necessary. So, we proceeded to insert five Zephyr valves into the segmental bronchi of the right upper and middle lobes.

A double-lumen endotracheal tube is then placed, and the patient is positioned for RIGHT robotic-assisted surgery.

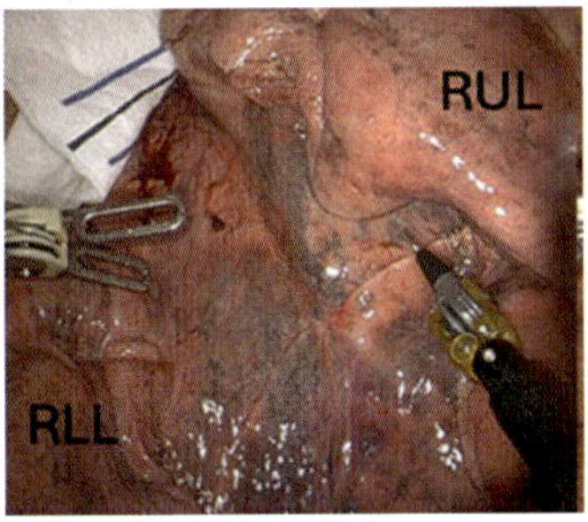

Surprisingly, the interlobar fissure on the RIGHT appeared to be nearly complete. Robotic dissection with electrocautery was commenced to divide the fused major fissure.

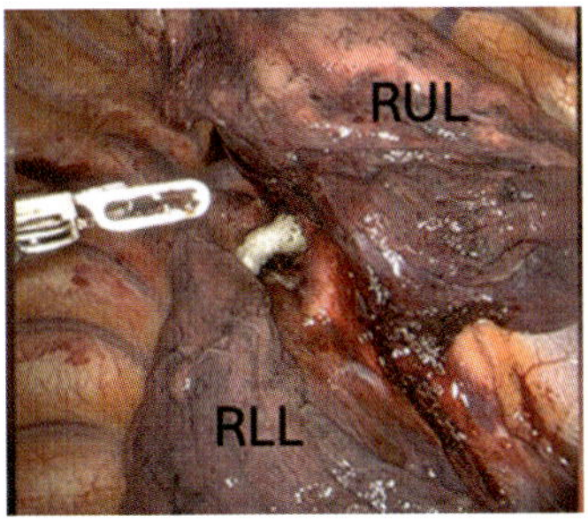

After careful dissection and stapling of the lung parenchyma, the interlobar fissure was completely divided.

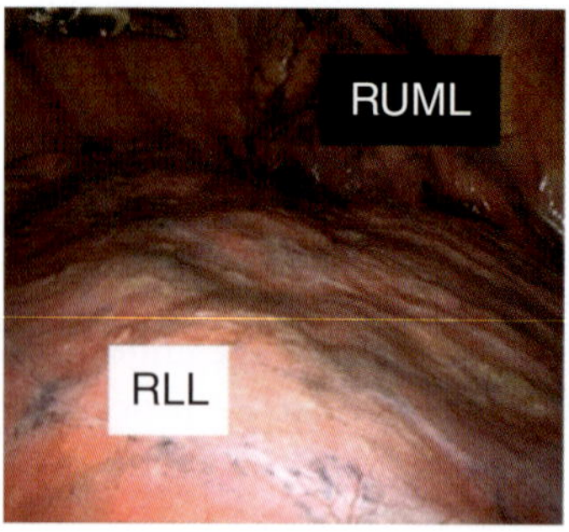

The right lung was then reventilated, but as the endobronchial valves were correctly functioning, only the right lower lobe re-expanded, leaving the right upper and middle lobes collapsed as verified by direct inspection.

And how did she do?

The patient had minimal postoperative air leak, and after a 72-hour observation period (as we would do after routine EBLVR to observe for pneumothorax), she returned home.

She has received a physiological and symptomatic improvement.

6.9 Conclusions

Not all patients suitable for LVR are suitable for EBLVR due to the presence of collateral ventilation. However, I believe it is reasonable to assess all patients for its presence and offer EBLVR to those who are negative. There is no evidence to suggest that the outcome from EBLVR is any worse than LVRS, but if all goes well, the hospital stay is less. The patient must be fully informed of the risks of pneumothorax which may prolong the stay and valve dysfunction which may require readmission. I believe that in patients with a similar disease profile the risk of LVR is determined by the severity of emphysema rather than the approach to LVR.

References

1 Criner GJ, Cordova F, Sternberg AL, Martinez FJ. The National Emphysema Treatment Trial (NETT) part II: lessons learned about lung volume reduction surgery. Am J Respir Crit Care Med. 2011;184(8):881–893.

2 Criner GJ, Sue R, Wright S, Dransfield M, Rivas-Perez H, Wiese T, et al. A multicenter randomized controlled trial of zephyr endobronchial valve treatment in heterogeneous emphysema (LIBERATE). Am J Respir Crit Care Med. 2018;198(9):1151–1164.

3 Hayanga JWA, Luo X, Reddy S, Mehaffey JH, Rothenberg P, Chauhan D, et al. Endobronchial valve therapy vs lung volume reduction surgery in the United States. Ann Thorac Surg. 2025; S0003-4975(25):00663-0.

4 Lee M, Dhanji AR, Perikleous P, Baranowski R, Lau KKW, Waller D. Bronchoscopic lung volume reduction as the treatment of choice versus robotic-assisted lung volume reduction surgery in similar patients with emphysema – an initial experience of the benefits and complications. Int J Chron Obstruct Pulmon Dis. 2024;19:1021–1032.

5 Mulryan K, Sorensen J, Waller D, Redmond K. Lung volume reduction surgery: a micro-costing analysis from a national tertiary referral centre. Eur J Cardiothorac Surg. 2024;65(6):ezae222.

6 Buttery SC, Banya W, Bilancia R, Boyd E, Buckley J, Greening NJ, et al. Lung volume reduction surgery versus endobronchial valves: a randomised controlled trial. Eur Respir J. 2023;61(4):2202063.

7 Valipour A, Slebos DJ, Herth F, Darwiche K, Wagner M, Ficker JH, et al. Endobronchial valve therapy in patients with homogeneous emphysema. Results from the IMPACT study. Am J Respir Crit Care Med. 2016;194(9):1073–1082.

8 Wahidi MM, Lentz RJ, Criner GJ, Gompelmann D, Ing AJ, Kapp CM, et al. Bronchoscopic lung volume reduction with endobronchial valves: a consensus statement on practical aspects of patient selection and periprocedural management. Respiration. 202515:1–24.

9 Shafiq M, Polhemus E, Perkins R, Forth V, Marshall MB. Bilateral bronchoscopic lung volume reduction after surgical fissure completion. Chest. 2022;162(2):e73–e75.

10 Majid A, Kheir F, Alape D, Chee A, Parikh M, DeVore L, et al. Combined thoracoscopic surgical stapling and endobronchial valve placement for lung volume reduction with incomplete lobar fissures: an experimental pilot animal study. J Bronchology Interv Pulmonol. 2020;27(2):128–134.

11 Lui A, Alam N, Cheung F, Wright G. The cove study—phase I study of VATS fissure completion prior to endobronchial valve insertion for severe COPD patients with collateral ventilation (COVE). Heart Lung Circ. 2025;34:S6.

12 Combined Zephyr Valve System with Inter-lobar Fissure Completion for Lung Volume Reduction in Emphysema: A Pilot Randomized Controlled Trial. 2021. https://clinicaltrials.gov/study/NCT04801108

7

Complications of Lung Volume Reduction

7.1 Lung Volume Reduction Surgery

7.1.1 Persistent Air Leak

Surgeon: What would be your definition of a "persistent" air leak?

Pulmonologist: I would say longer than seven days.

But are there any particular factors that might influence your definition?

Yes, I suppose the condition of the underlying lung, so those with more diffuse, severe emphysema may be expected to have a more prolonged leak.

What about the leak itself?

I guess a large volume leak or one that was increasing, not reducing, would indicate earlier intervention. Also. If the remaining lung is collapsed or if the patient is decompensating.

I agree, and I think the last factor is one of the most important. A large air leak may cause the patient to desaturate on minimal exercise, but the prolonged presence of a drain will also cause immobility, increase the risk of pneumonia and pleural infection.

How long do you wait before intervening in the postoperative period?

In general, I think that there is a tendency to wait too long before re-intervention. There is always the concern about the risk of further general anaesthesia, but the longer the patient remains immobile, the greater the risk. I would be influenced by the volume and pattern of leak and the expansion of the lung and reoperate within 72 hours if needed.

What if the lung was expanded and the air leak was less than 1000 ml/min?

I think then there is a case for closed pleurodesis via the drain. Talc slurry is most likely to cause pleural adhesions, but it can be painful and may further compromise the patient's respiratory function. Autologous blood pleurodesis is therefore probably the best alternative.

What about endobronchial valve insertion?

I would probably not advise that approach in this situation after LVRS. If the patient is going to have another general anaesthetic (as most surgeons require for endobronchial LVR [EBLVR]), then surgical closure of the leak is to be preferred. If the leak is coming from the target lobe, then by definition, the fact that the patient needed LVRS means that there is collateral ventilation, so valves can never completely stop the leak. If the leak is coming from the non-target lobe, then the same applies and one assumes that that lobe is the better perfused and most important in terms of function.

What if the anaesthetist was concerned about the risk of a further general anaesthetic if the patient's respiratory condition was worsening?

Then, I guess I would ask you to consider endobronchial valve insertion under spontaneous ventilation. But I would ask you to observe the following steps:

1. **Check that the drain is secured tightly and that there is no obvious leak around the drain.**
2. **First occlude the main bronchus with the balloon to ensure that the air leak is actually coming from the lung – if the air leak persists when the bronchus is occluded, then have courage and remove the drain when the lung is expanded again.**
3. **Inflate the balloon in the lobar bronchi and then in the segmental bronchi or even subsegmental bronchi, and observe the air leak for reduction or cessation.**
4. **A more ingenuous method has been suggested using the Chartis® system. With the drain on suction, the balloon connected to the Chartis® catheter is inserted into the bronchi as above. In the lobar bronchus, the pressure trace will show the patient's inspiratory pressure overlapped together with the negative pressure from the drain suction.**
5. **When the balloon occludes the segment where the main leak arises, the trace will just show the negative pressure of the suction theoretically conducted through the alveolar-pleural fistula [1].**

Does the way you manage the chest drains affect the duration of postoperative air leak?

7.1.2 Suction or Not?

If the lung can expand to fill the pleural space, then enough suction to obtain pleural apposition between visceral and parietal surfaces may hasten the resolution of the leak by the formation of adhesions.

If the remaining lung will not fill the pleural space, then drainage will create a pressure gradient across the parenchyma and potentially open junctions between alveolar epithelia, allowing air from the subpleural alveolar spaces to escape into the pleural cavity. Further application or increased suction will just potentiate this pressure-dependent air leak [2].

7.1.3 Digital Drainage vs Underwater Seal

Is there any benefit from investing in digital drainage systems after LVRS?

There may be some benefit in using a digital drainage system over a water seal in order to give a more objective evaluation of the size of the leak or to visualize trends [3].

In reality, their main benefit is to allow mobility whilst maintaining suction, but if one does not want added negative pressure, then it may be cheaper to use an underwater seal system or even a flutter valve drainage bag, which actually may be more efficient than a bottle and underwater seal [4].

And its use may enable earlier discharge from the hospital.

7.1.4 Subcutaneous Emphysema

Often associated with a persistent, high-volume air leak, subcutaneous emphysema is a collection of air under the skin. Its incidence may be as common as around 1 in 50 thoracic operations [5].

Its sudden appearance is certainly shocking for many inexperienced or non-surgical staff and quite frightening for the patient and their family.

That's right, but the cosmetic consequences are far worse than any immediate physiological danger in this post-lung resection situation. The frequently expressed fear of the need for endotracheal intubation to treat impending laryngeal compression is misplaced.

How do you suggest we treat the situation? I have seen various drainage procedures employed.

In the presence of an indwelling drain, it indicates that the rate of air leak exceeds the rate of drainage. Either the source of the leak has increased,

or the method of drainage is inadequate. The management, therefore, either requires control of the source or an increase in the drainage. The former may require operative intervention or endobronchial occlusion. The latter may involve increasing the suction on the drainage. However, flow rate is more effectively increased by increasing the diameter of the drainage tubes. Thus, either the existing drain can be replaced with a drain of greater calibre, or a second drain of larger calibre should be inserted.

But even these measures may not prevent spreading of the existing subcutaneous air with increasing distress to all concerned.

Ok, well, this can be addressed more directly by the insertion of a subcutaneous drain, which does not need an underwater seal! Suction can be applied, but it may just lead to drain occlusion. When the drain is removed, the stab wound for insertion should be left open and covered with a loose dressing.

Historically, was it not the practice just to make anterior chest stab wounds into the subcutaneous tissue?

Certainly, this method can still be used with the application of a suction device (VAC device) to the wound [6].

When would you consider re-operating?

This decision should be primarily guided by the clinical condition of the patient because simple chest radiography may be difficult to interpret in the presence of a large amount of subcutaneous air. Thoracic CT may be required to assess lung re-expansion.

In some circumstances, there are patchy adhesions to a previous incision. In this situation, the lung may not be able to re-expand fully, and leaking air will be directed out of the pleural space through the potential defect in the chest wall tissues. The fastest way to remedy this problem is to reoperate, divide the adhesions and control the source of the air leak [7].

How can postoperative subcutaneous emphysema be avoided?

By attention to detail in chest drainage. Firstly, if there is a risk for a large air leak, as in LVRS for severe emphysema, then an adequate size drain or number of drains should be used. Tunnelling the drain can be used to reduce the possibility of a peri-tubular leak, and care should be taken to accurately close the subcutaneous tissues as well as the skin around the drain. Secondly, the flow of air should be free of obstruction further distal to the site of drain insertion. Kinking of the drain should be avoided, and suction equipment should be checked that it is functioning, or it will act as an effective block to the flow.

7.1.5 Mediastinal Emphysema (Pneumomediastinum)

Is this finding a medical emergency?

Certainly not in the context of a postoperative air leak after LVRS. If one can exclude the more dramatic causes of oesophageal rupture or rupture of a major airway, then the finding just indicates a subpleural escape of the air leak. It should be managed in a similar way to subcutaneous emphysema by ensuring adequate pleural drainage or re-operation to close the leak.

So mediastinal drainage?

Definitely NOT. In this context, the only danger from tension is from the pleural cavity, so pleural drainage is indicated if there is associated pneumothorax.

7.1.6 Drain Removal

After LVRS, when can you safely remove the drains? Presumably, after a certain period of observation, once the air leak has stopped.

In most straightforward cases, but once the leak persists for longer than 7 days, one can consider removing the drain even if there is still an apparent leak.

I would be very scared of the consequences of removing a bubbling drain.

Yes, I can appreciate your trepidation, but you are assuming that the air leak is coming from the parenchyma of the lung and that, without drainage, a tension pneumothorax would rapidly develop with danger to the patient.

Where else would the air leak be coming from?

7.1.7 Entrained Air

There may be entrainment of air around the drain due to the negative intrathoracic pressures generated during respiration. This will be more likely after prolonged drainage, where an inflammatory track may have formed around the tube, and in thinner patients, where tissue closure may be inadequate and may not form a seal around the drain.

This is surely just a theoretical argument.

Not necessarily, it should be possible to differentiate between entrained room air and expired gas from the lung.

How so?

Entrained air will have a lower CO_2 tension than expired air. Thus, simple analysis by capnography may differentiate between the two sources. If the capnograph waveform does not follow the characteristic pattern with respiration, then the drain air is entrained, and the drain can be removed. Chest drain units with in-built CO_2 detectors may also be used [8, 9].

But surely, in most cases, the air leak is actually coming from the lung parenchyma?

7.1.8 Pressure-dependent Air Leak

True, but in many cases of an apparent persistent air leak, the drainage mechanism is in itself perpetuating the leak. This is a pressure-dependent air leak, which may occur if the lung cannot expand to fill the pleural space due to a thickened inflammatory cortex or an actual size mismatch between the previously hyperexpanded rib cage and the resected emphysematous lung, i.e. after LVRS.

How can one recognize this pressure-dependent air leak?

This air leak may only be seen on coughing and may cease when suction is removed from the drainage system, i.e. when the parenchymal-pleural pressure gradient is reduced.

So, what action would you take to prove the point?

If this phenomenon is suspected, then by opening the bubbling drain to the atmosphere, the negative pressure promoting the leak is removed. If the lung is trapped due to the development of a chronic visceral cortex, then it will remain stable when the drain is disconnected.

But the patient should be kept under close observation.

Of course, and a repeat chest X-ray was taken to confirm no change in the lung expansion before drain removal.

This sounds to me like a very rare clinical occurrence.

Well, sorry to shock you, but in a series of over 200 prolonged air leaks after partial lung resection, 80% were found to be pressure dependent and the drain could be removed. Only one patient required re-operation [10].

Instead of opening the drain to air, could you not just clamp the drain?

7.1.9 Provocative Clamping

In the presence of significant entrainment of air around the drain, clamping may actually make the situation worse, particularly if the lung is not entrapped. In this case, air can enter the pleural cavity, but its expulsion via the drain would be blocked, so either the lung may collapse further or the patient may develop subcutaneous emphysema.

If the lung is expanded and the air leak is barely visible or reading <100 ml/min on a digital system, then it is not unreasonable to clamp the drain. This assumes that there is an element of pressure-dependency to the air leak. One must carefully observe the patient's condition and repeat a chest X-ray after an interval of two to four hours to assess any development of a pneumothorax in the event of a true parenchymal, pressure-independent leak [11].

7.2 Endobronchial Valves

7.2.1 Elective Complication: Non-response

How many patients do not feel they have had a good response from EBLVR? I would hope that having gone through the detailed selection process that having gone through the detailed selection very few would not feel a benefit.

Unfortunately, a non-response rate of 30% is reported [12].

How do you define non-response to EBLVR?

Basically, the non-responders can be separated into those who have no symptomatic benefit but have target lobe collapse and those who do not. For definitive purposes, satisfactory collapse has been defined as a target lobe volume reduction of more than 50% or a residual target lobe volume of less than 350 ml.

Personally, I think that one should not accept a sub-optimal result and that less than total lobar collapse necessitates further investigation. And why would there be non-response if lobar collapse and volume reduction were achieved?

There are two main reasons: firstly, the target lobe may be well perfused, causing a significant pulmonary arteriovenous shunt and resultant hypoxia, which may not be apparent until the patient begins to exercise. The second reason may be that the patient's dyspnoea was not due primarily to disrupted mechanics from hyperinflation. Other lung diseases or cardiac causes may be the main contributory factors.

There is also the possibility that successful and fast target lobe collapse will result in redirection of tidal volume to the most compliant areas in the rest of the lungs, particularly if there was significant bilateral disease and unilateral EBLVR was performed.

Why should this present a problem?

The resulting compensatory hyperinflation may not only cause recurrent problems with deranged chest wall mechanics but may also worsen any ventilation: perfusion mismatch with resulting hypoxia and breathlessness, as illustrated in Case Study 1.

Is this not an argument for targeted LVRS rather than lobar EBLVR!

Or, more provocatively, an argument for one-stage bilateral EBLVR?

And what about those in whom lobar collapse is not obtained?

The most common cause, in just over half of the patients, is valve obstruction due to granulation tissue (Figure 7.1) or thickened sputum. Then, common causes include incorrect valve sizing, allowing for paravalvular leaks, or valves being held open due to oversizing. Rarely, valves may be expectorated if not fitted correctly (Figure 7.2).

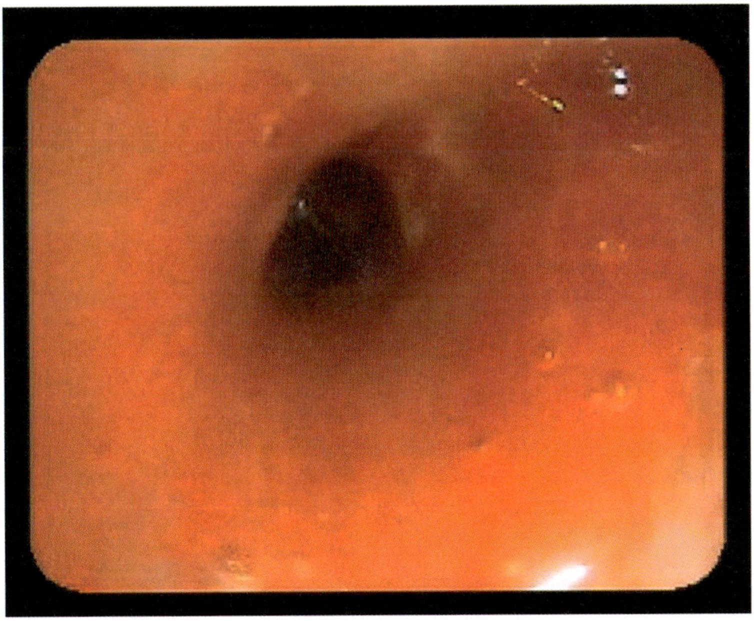

Figure 7.1 Endobronchial valve occlusion by granulation tissue.

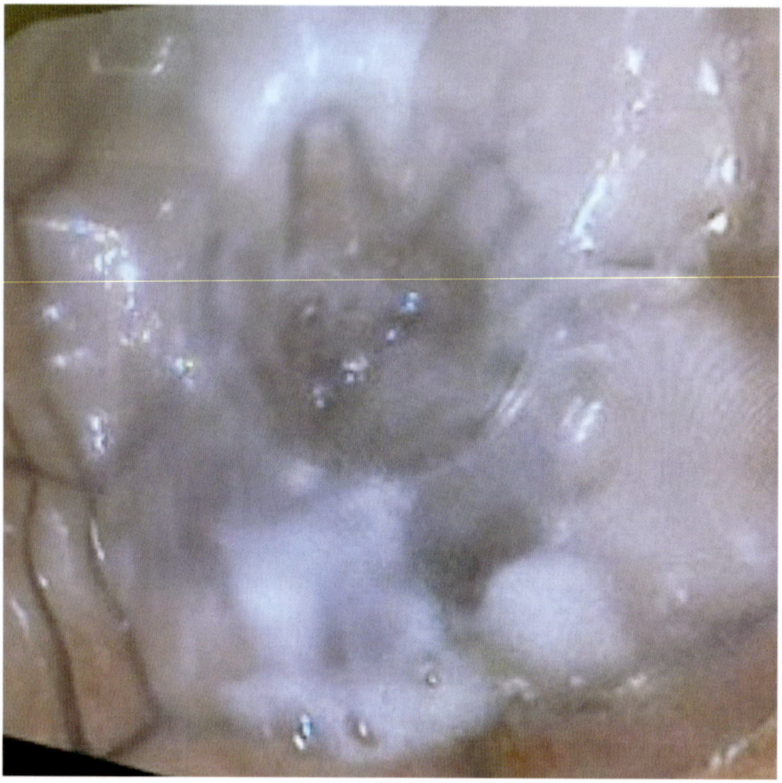

Figure 7.2 Endobronchial displacement – the Zephyr valve has inverted and embedded in an adjacent lobar bronchus.

No clinically relevant predictors for granulation tissue formation were identified.

So, all these can be fixed by repeated bronchoscopy and replacement or clearance?

Yes, in the majority, and the practitioner should have a low threshold for repeat bronchoscopy in the absence of any satisfactory response or loss of an initial good response. It is good practice to obtain a repeat CT with software analysis to target any open segmental bronchi previously missed, which require valve insertion. A malpositioned valve (size discrepancy or paravalvular leak) must be replaced, as should a valve blocked with granulation tissue. Sputum blockage is easily corrected with saline lavage.

So, there are some patients whose non-response cannot be explained?

However, there will remain a small proportion, probably less than 10%, who continue to have lobar inflation despite adequate valve placement. It has been thought that no further intervention was possible in these cases. Once all these measures have been addressed, then the possibility of occult collateral ventilation should be considered [13]. Repeat the Chartis assessment with the valves in situ is possible and may be informative and definitive.

In these cases, would you offer LVRS to the target lobe?

That is the standard treatment.

Presumably, then you would remove the unsuccessful valves?

Not necessarily. I have had successful results from sequential LVRS after EBLVR without removing them. Assuming there is no concern about bacterial valve colonization.

Are you not concerned about future valve complications, including blockage?

Not if one considers maximizing the effectiveness of the in-dwelling valves by leaving them in situ and considering fissure division rather than LVRS (Case Study 2), as we discussed in Chapter 6. Even if the valves become blocked in the long term, the lobe collapses. Reinflation due to occult collateral ventilation (CV) is impossible if the fissure is completely divided. If reinflation did occur later, then it must be attributable to valve displacement and thus remedied by valve replacement.

Whilst fissure division rather than standard LVRS remains experimental, its evaluation in this population of non-responders to EBLVR seems the most appropriate subject.

Indeed, and there are existing studies in progress [14].

7.2.2 Non-elective Complication: Post-procedural Pneumothorax

A spontaneous pneumothorax (SP) following EBLVR is not uncommon. It is reported to occur in around 30% of procedures in large series [15–17]. However, it is associated with successful lobar collapse, and therefore those who suffer post EBLVR-SP go on to have a real symptomatic benefit [16].

Can you predict who is most at risk from a post-EBLVR SP?

There are no validated criteria, but logically, the more severe the emphysema score in the non-target lobe and the greater the volume loss in the target lobe, the higher the risk of pneumothorax. The hypothesis is that a sudden redistribution of air flow causes rupture of an existing area of weakness in the non-target lobe visceral pleura.

Do pleural adhesions really cause post-EBLVR SP?

As I said, large volume shifts after successful EBLVR and subsequent repositioning of the lung could subsequently rupture the visceral pleura. A higher number and larger size of pleural adhesions in the treated lung were associated with a higher occurrence of pneumothorax after treatment [18].

May I contrarily suggest that the presence of adhesions just indicates previous sites of pneumothoraces? So, there is not a direct causal relationship with the adhesions but rather with a pre-existing site of pleural weakness.

If one could identify those at higher risk of SP, should one consider prophylactic chest drain insertion?

One group has begun placing a prophylactic 16 Fr chest drain on the side of EBLVR at the time of valve placement. The drain is placed on an ambulatory drainage system, and the patient is discharged. The drain is then removed in 7 days as an outpatient if there is no clinical or radiological evidence of an air leak [19].

But chest tube placement is not without risks of morbidity and mortality.

Absolutely, there are immediate risks at insertion of iatrogenic visceral injury and bleeding from introducing a drain into a pleural cavity with a hyperinflated lung, where there may be pleural adhesions.

These risks could be reduced by image (ultrasound) guided drain insertion or stopping ventilation if the procedure is performed under general anaesthesia.

That's true, but there is still the risk of longer-term problems with intercostal neuralgia and wound infection. So, I think that further randomized evidence is required before the benefits of prophylactic drainage are shown to outweigh the potential risks.

If you do not insert a prophylactic drain, how long do you think one should observe the patient after EBLVR?

In the LIBERATE trial, 93% of the pneumothoraces occurred within 13 days of bronchoscopy, but 76% occurred within the first 3 days, and the median onset time was 1 day post bronchoscopy procedure [15]. So I would advise observation until discharge on the morning of the third postoperative day.

That sounds fair, but the postoperative stay is frustrating for the patient and the hospital and is an area for further prospective research to compare the risks of delayed post EBLVR-SP with the benefits of earlier discharge.

I understand that some pulmonologists have suggested a method for reducing the risk of developing post EBLVR-SP?

Yes, they have. Working on the assertion that the gradual collapse of the target lobe reduces the rate of redistribution of ventilation and possibly the barotrauma to areas of weakness in the non-target lobe. A 2-stage protocol has been reported where, in the first procedure, all but the most proximal sub-segment of the targeted lobe is occluded, followed, one month later, by the bronchus of the last subsegment. The pneumothorax rate was reduced to 12.5% [20].

The theory makes sense, but again, it would be necessary for two post-EBLVR observation periods and further use of hospital resources. Further prospective, comparative results are awaited, but these should be targeted on the most at risk population. And this is the area where initial research should be directed.

Well, I understand that further studies are needed in this matter but surely the management is more straightforward.

Not so fast. I think that we need to discuss a slightly controversial area surrounding this problem. Patients with these pneumothoraces are rarely stable and can deteriorate quickly, so one should have a low threshold for drainage. We have discussed how long to persist with drainage of a post-LVRS air leak, but how would you manage a persistent air leak in these patients post-EBLVR?

If the air leak persists for more than 72 hours with a high volume of more than 1000 mL/min, then I would consider removing one or more of the valves as per current recommendations [21]. In the LIBERATE trial, 1 in 3 of those needing drainage of a post-EBLVR pneumothorax required the removal of at least one valve.

What do you think is the benefit of doing this?

I suppose that if the pneumothorax is caused by a sudden redistribution of the tidal volume from the collapsed target lobe to the non-target lobe, then by removing the valves, the flow to the site of the leak will be reduced. Also, re-expansion of the target lobe may help to close the air leak by promoting pleural adhesions.

But how does that leave the patient? Surely, they will lose any benefit of volume reduction and will require a third procedure to re-insert the valves. But furthermore, they will still be at risk of a second post-EBLVR pneumothorax, and so the cycle could begin again.

Are you suggesting an alternative plan?

I am. I suggest that if the air leak lasts for longer than 72 hours, then surgical closure with a minimally invasive approach should be performed (Case Study 3).

Is that not putting the patient at considerable risk from a further general anaesthetic?

That has been used as a reason to pursue non-operative treatment, unless one believes that some patients may be fit for EBLVR but not LVRS, the risks of long-term drainage and the need for a further LVR procedure are probably greater.

When one operates, where is the leak usually seen?

It is invariably from a bleb or bulla in the non-target lobe (usually the apex of the lower lobe in upper lobe EBLVR), which may or may not be surrounded by pleural adhesions.

Finally, just to continue the controversy. One should consider that one may not need to drain a post-EBLVR pneumothorax. In the LIBERATE trial, 17% of those who developed a pneumothorax did not require chest tube placement.

How do you explain the pneumothorax in those cases?

After EBLVR, some patients may develop non-expandable lung physiology and a size-mismatch between the remaining lung and the previously hyperexpanded chest cavity after successful lobar collapse, causing pneumothorax *ex vacuo* [22].

It may be necessary to drain the initial event on clinical grounds, but if the lung fails to expand, then this phenomenon should be considered.

Indeed, air leaks into the pleural space without visceral pleural injury but from deformation of subpleural alveolar units, resulting in the transient opening of alveolar–pleural fistulas. Pleural manometry proximal to an occluded drain may help to differentiate a pressure-dependent from a pressure-independent pneumothorax.

7.3 CASE STUDY 1: Compensatory Hyperinflation as a Complication of EBLVR

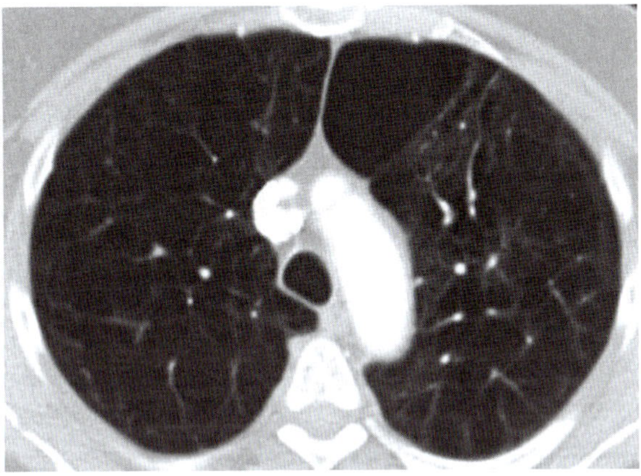

This 57-year-old female was thought to be an ideal candidate for EBLVR. She was significantly hyperinflated (RV 193% predicted) and was of relatively low risk (FEV_1 800 mL, 31% predicted, BMI 22 kg/m^2, DLCO 29% predicted). She had bilateral upper lobe targets on the CT emphysema score and quantitative lung perfusion. Her Chartis assessment for collateral ventilation was negative.

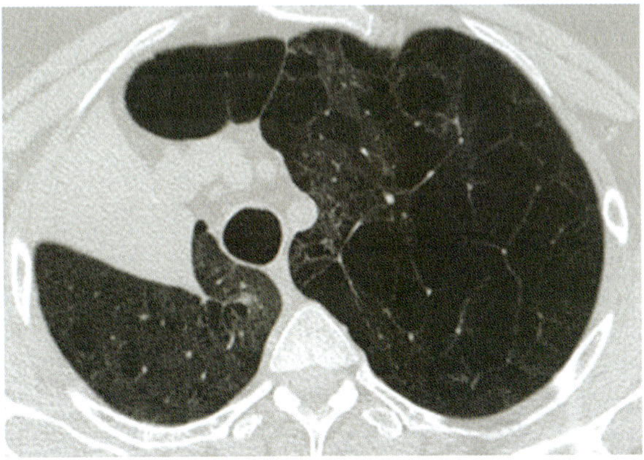

Right upper lobe EBLVR was performed with a good response and right upper lobar collapse.

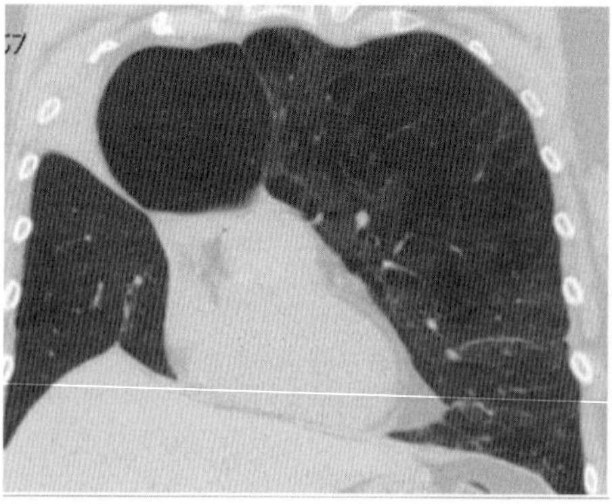

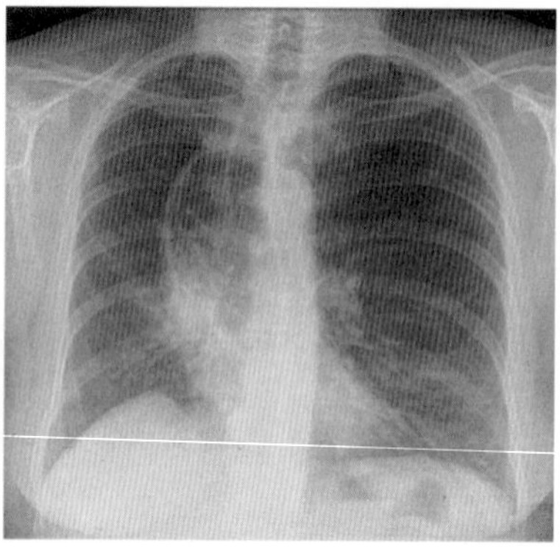

At 6 months after the procedure, she was more breathless than at baseline. She remained hyperinflated: RV 180% predicted, and her lung function had worsened: FEV_1 680 ml/min, 27% predicted, DLCO 29% predicted.

The patient had suffered **compensatory hyperinflation** of the bullous left upper lobe.

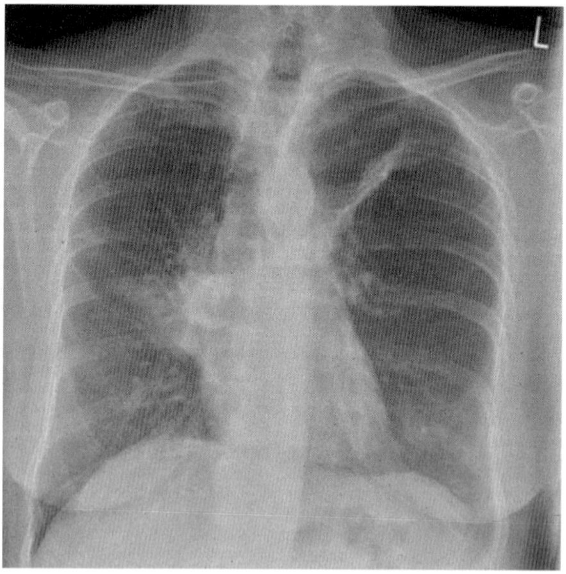

The patient underwent left upper lobe LVRS with significant symptomatic improvement.

7.4 CASE STUDY 2: Interlobar Fissure Division in Non-responder to EBLVR

This 71-year-old female fulfilled the selection criteria for volume reduction. She was very hyperinflated (RV 288% predicted), had significant airways obstruction (FEV_1 740 ml/min, 35% predicted) and preserved gas exchange (DLCO 39% predicted).

SUMMARY

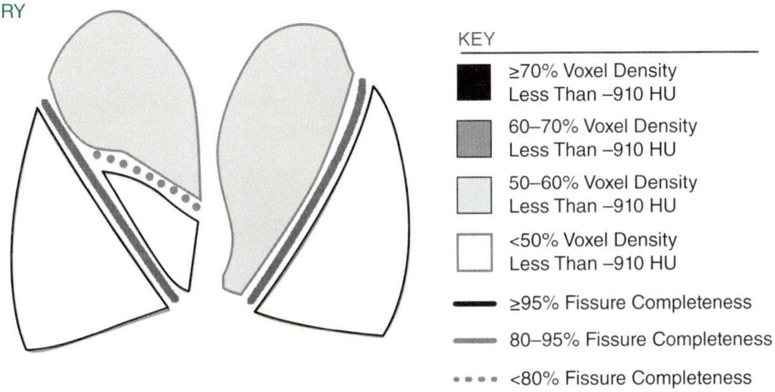

RESULTS

	RIGHT LUNG				LEFT LUNG	
	RUL	RUL + RML	RML	RLL	LUL	LLL
% Fissure Completeness	70.1	91.4	72.9	91.4	92.3	92.3
% Voxel Density Less Than –910 HU	52	50	37	31	51	35
% Voxel Density Less Than –950 HU	32	30	16	14	30	18
Inspiratory Volume (ml)	1483	1732	249	1367	1341	1213

Her CT suggested a left upper lobe target and a sufficiently complete left major fissure to consider EBLVR.

She underwent Chartis balloon catheter assessment with no evidence of collateral ventilation, and five left endobronchial valves were inserted.

Unfortunately, despite an initial symptomatic improvement, the patient soon deteriorated with a mMRC dyspnoea score of 4. Her lung function tests had improved: FEV_1 1.02 l (47% predicted), but she remained hyperinflated with RV 180% predicted and had only partial radiological left upper collapse.

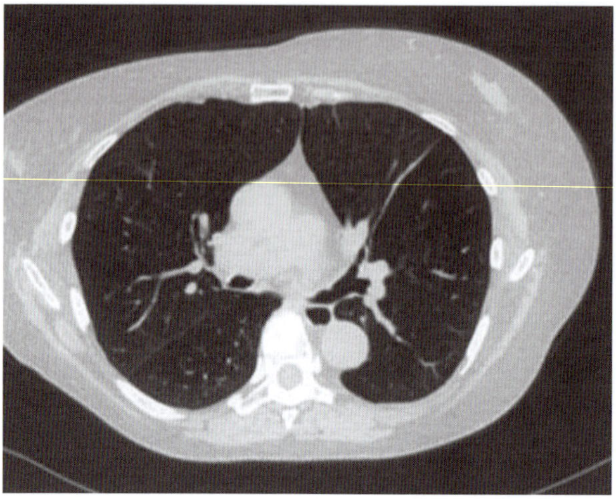

She underwent revisional bronchoscopy with replacement of one valve, which was suboptimally sited.

SUB-SEGMENT	VALVE PLACEMENT LOCATION
LB1 + 2a	LB1 + 2a
LB1 + 2b	LB1 + 2b
LB3a	LB3
LB3b	LB3
LB4a	LB4
LB4b	LB4
LB5a	LB5
LB5b	LB5
Quantity of Valves Observed	5

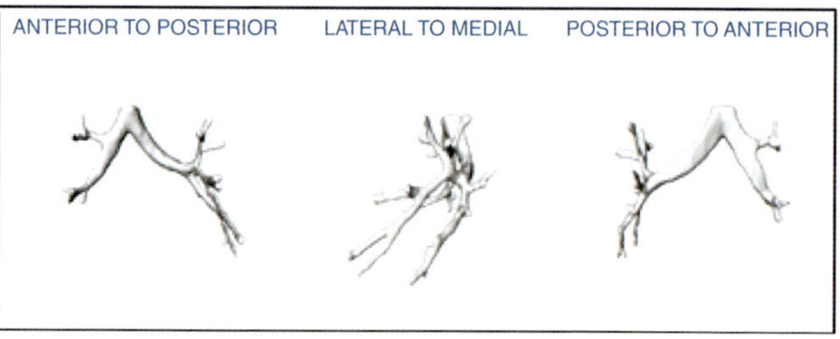

Repeat CT software analysis confirmed satisfactory valve placement but a target lung volume reduction (TLVR) of only 56%.

She then proceeded to left robotic interlobar fissure division. The fissure was more incomplete than predicted from the StratX assessment, but intraoperative left upper lobe collapse was obtained.

Postoperative recovery was uncomplicated, with postoperative left upper lobe collapse and symptomatic improvement.

7.5 CASE STUDY 3: Post-EBLVR Pneumothorax

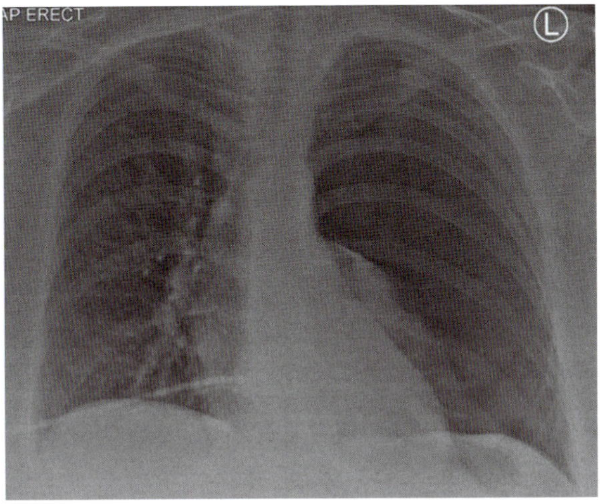

This patient had immediate target lobe collapse after left upper lobe EBLVR, but complained of chest pain and breathlessness, and began to desaturate within a few hours of the procedure.

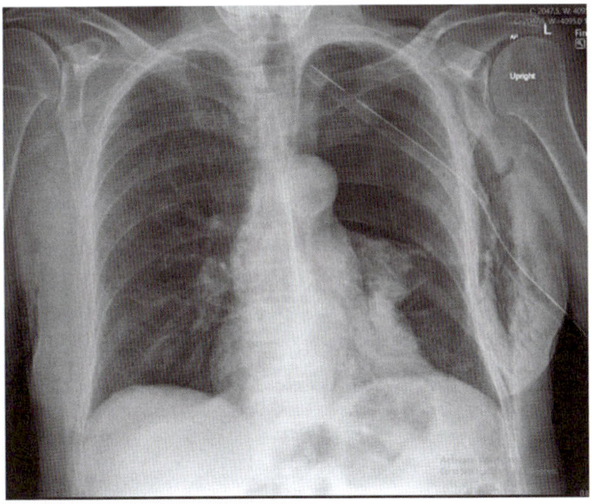

A left intercostal chest drain was inserted with symptomatic and clinical improvement.

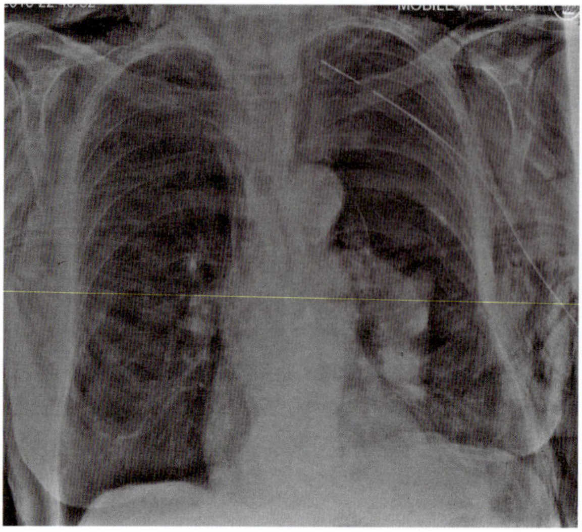

The patient had a persistent, high-volume air leak after three days of intercostal drainage and was developing subcutaneous emphysema. Left VATS exploration was performed.

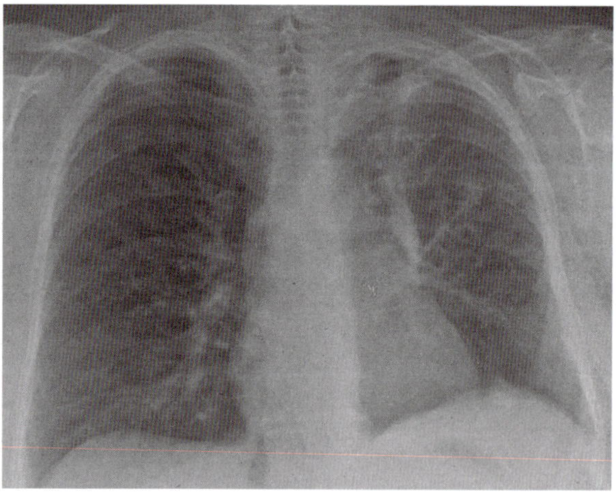

VATS stapled closure of the source of air leak from bullous emphysema in the apex of the non-target left lower lobe was successful, and the patient was discharged without a drain 48 hours later.

SUMMARY

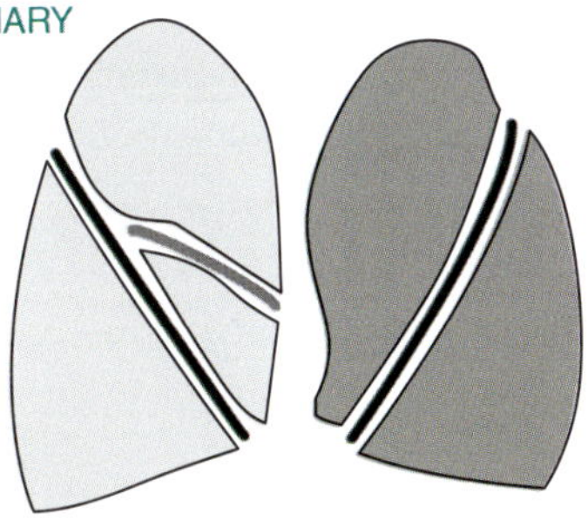

KEY

- ≥70% Voxel Density Less Than –910 HU
- 60–70% Voxel Density Less Than –910 HU
- 50–60% Voxel Density Less Than –910 HU
- <50% Voxel Density Less Than –910 HU
- ≥95% Fissure Completeness
- 80–95% Fissure Completeness
- <80% Fissure Completeness

RESULTS

	RIGHT LUNG				LEFT LUNG	
	RUL	RUL + RML	RML	RLL	LUL	LLL
% Fissure Completeness	95.6	100.0	96.5	100.0	100.0	100.0
% Voxel Density Less Than –910 HU	53	52	50	59	60	61
% Voxel Density Less Than –950 HU	23	21	16	33	28	29
Inspiratory Volume (ml)	1670	2340	670	1560	2144	2047

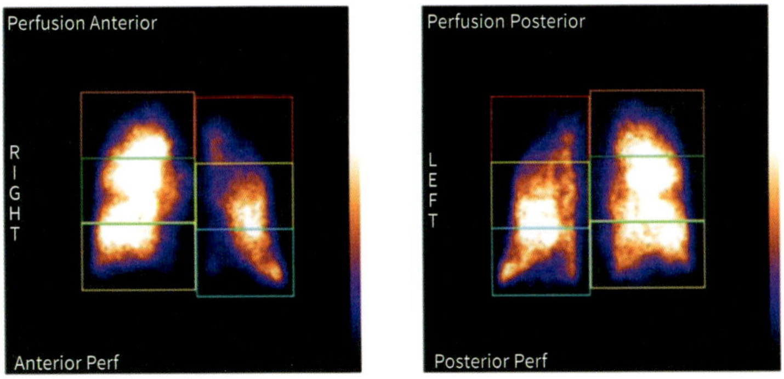

	Perfusion% Geometric Mean		Ventilation%	
	Right	Left	Right	Left
Upper	13.3	6.1		
Middle	30.5	18.1		
Lower	18.5	13.5		
Total	**62.3**	**37.7**		

This patient had several risk factors for developing a post-EBLVR-SP: a complete major fissure; a high emphysema score in the non-target lobe; a large volume in the target left upper lobe and relative homogeneity, on both emphysema and perfusion scores, with little interlobar difference on the target side.

7.6 Conclusions

LVRS

The best time to treat a postoperative air leak is while the patient is still on the operating table. Work with the anaesthetist to check for leaks on re-ventilation before extubation and have a low threshold for further lung stapling. Once the patient has returned to the ward, a desire to return to surgery for a further air leak is laudable, but one must be aware of the potential risks from a second general anaesthetic in a short time period in a patient with severe COPD. There is also the danger of playing "whack-a-mole" with the air leak, as closing one in the fragile lung may only precipitate another elsewhere.

In the postoperative management it is worth remembering that after LVRS the chest wall remodels to meet the lung, rather than the remaining lung expanding to fill the cavity, and this process may take several days. Sometimes this may not occur fully, and a residual space may be left which will not respond to increased suction or prolonged drainage.

EBLVR

If one is happy that valve placement is optimal, then do not accept second-best in the postoperative course. If total target lobe collapse has not been achieved within 72 hours or if initial collapse is subsequently lost, then be prepared to re-investigate. Revision bronchoscopy should be undertaken irrespective of CT analysis, but occult CV may be present due to delayed opening of the low-resistance Channels of Martin. If this is suspected, then surgical intervention should be considered.

Post EBLVR pneumothorax should not be looked upon as a bad outcome. It usually follows immediate lobar collapse and is associated with a good long-term result. I believe that prompt surgical intervention to close the air leak is the most direct treatment and will reduce hospital stays. However, it is logistically easier to instigate if both EBLVR and LVRS are offered by an integrated team.

References

1 Tian Q, Qi F, An Y, Liu XC, Chen LA. Using the Chartis system to selectively target a lung segment with a persistent air leak. Eur Respir J. 2013 Jun;41(6):1461–1463.

2 Chopra A, Doelken P, Hu K, Huggins JT, Judson MA. Pressure-dependent pneumothorax and air leak: physiology and clinical implications. Chest. 2023 Sep;164(3):796–805.

3 Dooms CA, De Leyn PR, Yserbyt J, Decaluwe H, Ninane V. Endobronchial valves for persistent postoperative pulmonary air leak: accurate monitoring and functional implications. Respiration. 2012;84(4):329–333.

4 Waller DA, Edwards JG, Rajesh PB. A physiological comparison of flutter valve drainage bags and underwater seal systems for postoperative air leaks. Thorax. 1999 May;54(5):442–443.

5 Boulemden A, Aifesehi P, Pajaniappane A, Lau K, Bajaj A, Nakas A, et al. Subcutaneous drain insertion in patients with post-operative extensive subcutaneous surgical emphysema: a single centre experience. Gen Thorac Cardiovasc Surg. 2013;61(12):707–710.

6 Brown SW, Ison TJ, Holko MJ, Bahl N. Surgical blowhole incision for acute subcutaneous emphysema: a novel approach with negative-pressure wound therapy. Cureus. 2025 Oct 2;17(10):e93733.

7 Cerfolio RJ, Bryant AS, Maniscalco LM. Management of subcutaneous emphysema after pulmonary resection. Ann Thorac Surg. 2008 May;85(5):1759–1763; discussion 1764–1765.

8 Oparka JD, Walker WS. The application of capnography to differentiate peri-chest tube air leak from parenchymal leak following pulmonary surgery. Ann Cardiothorac Surg. 2014 Mar;3(2):219–220.

9 Cannone G, Campisi A, Comacchio GM, Lorenzoni G, Terzi S, Pangoni A, et al. Is chest tube capnography effective in differentiating between true and false air leaks after minimally invasive thoracic surgery? Gen Thorac Cardiovasc Surg. 2024 Nov;72(11):726–731.

10 Chopra A, Hu K, Judson MA, Fabian T, Nabagiez JP, Feustel PJ, et al. Association between drainage-dependent prolonged air leak after partial lung resection and clinical outcomes: a prospective cohort study. Ann Am Thorac Soc. 2022 Mar;19(3):389–398.

11 Cerfolio RJ, Minnich DJ, Bryant AS. The removal of chest tubes despite an air leak or a pneumothorax. Ann Thorac Surg. 2009 Jun;87(6):1690–1694; discussion 1694–1696.

12 Roodenburg SA, Klooster K, Hartman JE, Koster TD, van Dijk M, Slebos DJ. Revision bronchoscopy after endobronchial valve treatment for emphysema:

indications, findings and outcomes. Int J Chron Obstruct Pulmon Dis. 2021 Apr 21;16:1127–1136.

13 Koster TD, Shah PL, Valipour A, Criner GJ, Herth FJF, Sue R, et al. Optimizing clinical outcomes for bronchoscopic lung volume reduction with Zephyr® valves. Respir Med. 2024 Jun;227:107639.

14 Inter-lobar fissure completion as a salvage treatment in patients with failed bronchoscopic lung volume reduction 2022. https://clinicaltrials.gov/study/NCT05257681

15 Criner GJ, Sue R, Wright S, Dransfield M, Rivas-Perez H, Wiese T, et al. A Multicenter randomized controlled trial of zephyr endobronchial valve treatment in heterogeneous emphysema (LIBERATE). Am J Respir Crit Care Med. 2018 Nov 1;198(9):1151–1164.

16 Gompelmann D, Herth FJ, Slebos DJ, Valipour A, Ernst A, Criner GJ, et al. Pneumothorax following endobronchial valve therapy and its impact on clinical outcomes in severe emphysema. Respiration 2014;87:485–491.

17 Lee M, Dhanji AR, Perikleous P, Baranowski R, Lau KKW, Waller D. Bronchoscopic lung volume reduction as the treatment of choice versus robotic-assisted lung volume reduction surgery in similar patients with emphysema - an initial experience of the benefits and complications. Int J Chron Obstruct Pulmon Dis. 2024 May 9;19:1021–1032.

18 van Geffen WH, Klooster K, Hartman JE, Ten Hacken NHT, Kerstjens HAM, Wolf RFE, et al. Pleural Adhesion Assessment as a Predictor for Pneumothorax after Endobronchial Valve Treatment. Respiration. 2017;94(2):224–231.

19 Fitzmaurice GJ, Lau K, Redmond KC. The LIBERATE trial: options to reduce the risk of post-procedural pneumothorax and length of stay. Am J Respir Crit Care Med. 2018;198(12):1586–1587.

20 Egenod T, Guibert N, Ammar Y, Kessler R, Toublanc B, Favrolt N, et al. Endobronchial valves: 1st multicenter retrospective study on the 2-step approach. Respir Med Res. 2023;83:100957.

21 Herth FJF, Slebos DJ, Criner GJ, Valipour A, Sciurba F, Shah PL. Endoscopic lung volume reduction: an expert panel recommendation – update 2019. Respiration. 2019;97(6):548–557.

22 Hu K, S Benn B, Doelken P, Chopra A. The tale of two pneumothoraces after bronchoscopic lung volume reduction. Ann Am Thorac Soc. 2022;19(9):1596–1601.

8

Non-Lung Volume Reduction Surgery in Emphysema

8.1 Secondary Spontaneous Pneumothorax

Surgeon: You must admit many patients with secondary spontaneous pneumothorax (SSP) to emphysema during the year?

Physician: Indeed, apparently it is the commonest cause of spontaneous pneumothorax, with around 6000 patients per year admitted to hospital in England [1].

And they must present quite a burden to the hospital resources.

Quite, on average, the air leak duration is nearly 10 days in SSP [2], with this persistent air leak, leading to long hospital stays of 12–16 days [3, 4].

It is my impression that, considering those numbers, we don't get to operate on anywhere near that many patients.

That is definitely truc. A recent UK trial of ambulatory drainage of SSP found that only 7% of SSP patients proceeded to surgery to close the air leak [5].

Why do you think that is so few?

I am sure that there is a reluctance to consider surgery in this elderly population due to an underlying fear of the potential risk or morbidity and mortality. This is because many of the patients will be under the care of non-respiratory specialist physicians who may not be aware of the target population for lung volume reduction (LVR) or the selection criteria.

I am also afraid that these patients will be non-elective referrals to the thoracic surgery service, and therefore, the point of contact may be a trainee surgeon who, also, may not be aware of the type of patient who could benefit from surgery. They may have had little exposure to LVR surgery (LVRS) programmes themselves.

So, how can the principles of LVRS selection be applied to this population of patients who present with SSP?

Of course, in these patients with a persistent air leak, it is not possible to obtain contemporary lung function tests of dynamic and static lung volumes, but there may be recent historical results that may be of use. Failing that, these factors have been suggested in the most recent European Guidelines on the management of pneumothorax [6]: age, comorbidities, type of underlying lung disease, performance status, American Society of Anesthesiologists (ASA) score and degree of emphysema on computed tomography.

Furthermore, clinical examination and bedside echocardiography should exclude significant right heart failure, and blood gas analysis will indicate chronic hypercapnia.

Yes, these would be very informative.

If we judge the patient to be potentially suitable for surgery, when should we make the referral?

There is surprisingly little evidence-based information on the timing of surgical intervention in SSP. Historical data from the United Kingdom [7] and Norway [8] suggest a median time to resolution of air leak of nine days. More recent data from Singapore [3] suggest that 61% of air leaks resolve by seven days and 79% by 14 days, after which time resolution of air leaks proceeds at a much slower rate. So, intervention at seven days seems reasonable, suggesting surgical referral be made at five days [9] to allow for logistical considerations (transfer, operating availability).

What are the problems with waiting a little longer to refer?

Well, the risk of developing wound infection and/or pneumonia is significantly higher after seven days of chest tube treatment, independent of age [8], and importantly, more prolonged delays may decrease the effectiveness of thoracoscopy and increase the cost of care [10]. Thoracoscopic surgery has the benefits of lung function preservation in these patients [11].

We physicians may prefer closed pleurodesis via the chest tube in these elderly patients. Autologous blood pleurodesis (ABP) is favoured over talc as it is better tolerated and has been shown to be effective [12].

It is not so good for a larger air leak present throughout respiration [13], and I think that in SSP, there is a need for a sufficiently powered trial

evaluating the effect of ABP on short- and long-term clinical and economic outcomes, including pneumothorax recurrence rates.

We know that endobronchial valves have a role in LVR for emphysema and a role in post-resection air leak [14], so why not use EBV in SSP from emphysema?

Yes, there are early reports suggesting an efficacy of around 60% in resolving persistent air leaks of over 14 days duration [15]. Of course, there is the possibility of combining the benefits of LVR and reducing the air leak.

I have one question. How many valves can we insert? Should one try to completely control the leak or just diminish it to accelerate healing?

I think that it is informative to perform a Chartis® assessment first to check for CV.

But is that possible in the presence of an air leak?

Yes, it can be done in the non-target lobe and assess the major fissure or, as described in Chapter 7, the change in the trace may isolate the target segment. But if there is no CV, then the possibility of obtaining lobar collapse remains.

Can one risk lobar occlusion without prior assessment of lobar perfusion? Is there no risk of significant intrapulmonary shunting and consequent hypoxia?

There are several reassurances. One could rely on the lobar emphysema severity on the preoperative CT scan. One can also mimic the effect of lobar collapse with trial bronchial occlusion with the Chartis balloon catheter. Keep the balloon inflated for at least five minutes whilst ventilating on 28% oxygen. Observe any significant desaturation or hypotension, and in their absence, go for it.

Do you mean if Chartis is negative and no desaturation, go for lobar EBLVR with up to five segments occluded?

Why not? You may give the patient a "double whammy" of expedited discharge without a drain and the benefits of LVR.

8.2 Bullous Emphysema

Is there a difference between the surgical treatment of a bulla and LVR surgery? (Figure 8.1).

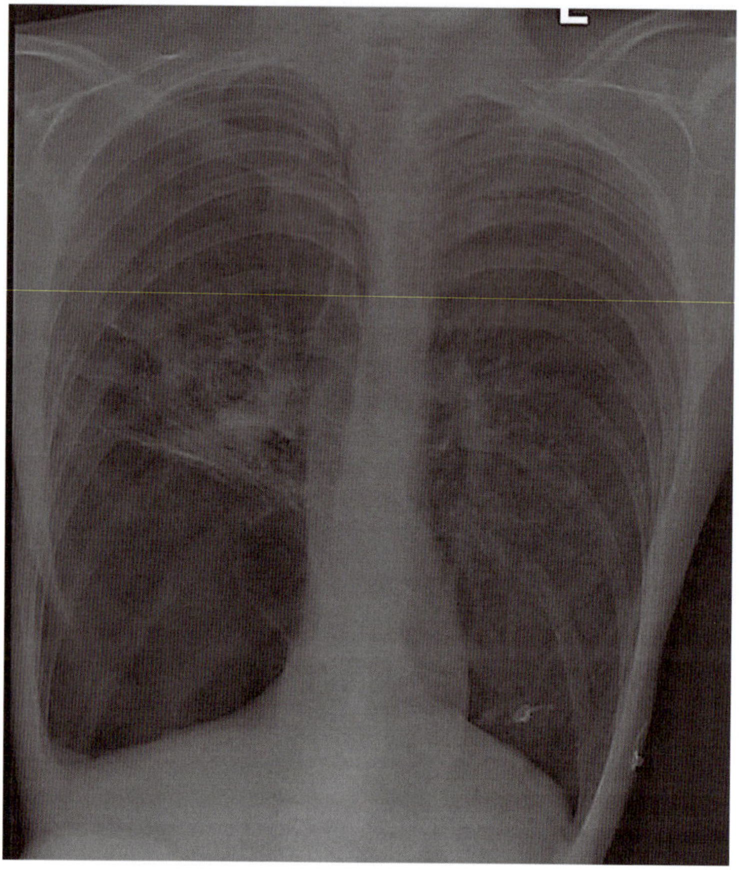

Figure 8.1 A patient with a large emphysematous bulla of the right lower lobe.

Not in principle. I view the division between bullectomy and LVRS as a false dichotomy. As discussed in Chapter 1, the physiology of an emphysematous bulla has often been misunderstood. The bulla is a well-localized area of non-functioning tissue, which is causing hyperinflation and relative under-ventilation of the surrounding lung tissue (but not by compression). There is no practical difference between a large bulla and a collection of smaller dilated air spaces (in diffuse emphysema).

So, is there any difference in the selection criteria for surgical intervention?

No, the bulla must be sufficiently large to be causing a deleterious effect on chest wall mechanics by hyperinflation and to be causing a significant ventilation:perfusion mismatch. So, the same physiological selection criteria apply regarding evidence of airways obstruction and preservation of diffusion capacity.

Does the surgical technique differ?

Yes, slightly. Because the target is more obvious. As we discussed in Chapter 1, the bulla expands because of the elastic recoil of the surrounding lung tissue, so this is of better quality than in the standard LVRS operation for diffuse emphysema. The margin for the stapled line is therefore more apparent. Also, in minimally invasive surgery, to facilitate exposure, the bulla can be punctured and deflated before resection, similar to deflating a hot-air balloon. It is possible to perform a bullectomy on a spontaneously ventilating patient if this deflation technique is used. As discussed in Chapter 4, there is little effect on oxygenation even if the bulla is opened.

Can you use endobronchial treatment for bullae?

Yes, there are reports of successful deflation of a large bulla in the right middle lobe by endobronchial occlusion [16, 17]. In another series, bullae in other lobes were deflated with a median of three valves, achieving physiological and functional improvements [18]. The main challenge in treating these patients is that it can prove challenging to identify the affected lung segment in order to treat a subsegment instead of the entire lobe. For the latter to be successful, there should be no interlobar collateral ventilation present [19]. I would just mention that this treatment has been taken to the extreme of "medical pneumonectomy" [20]. Multiple endobronchial valves were used to collapse the entire left "vanishing" lung! Not the approach I would advise.

Is percutaneous drainage of the bulla a therapeutic option?

Yes, in those cases where there may be a contraindication to surgical bullectomy, percutaneous drainage in conjunction with endobronchial valves [21] or the administration of intrabullous autologous blood [22] have been clinically successful.

I guess that this approach is also possible for an infected emphysematous bulla?

The primary treatment approach for this condition involves the prolonged administration of systemic antibiotics and close monitoring until recovery, which may take several weeks. If conservative management fails, bronchoscopic [23] or percutaneous [24] drainage can be considered.

So why isn't the percutaneous drainage method used more routinely instead of surgical bullectomy?

The Monaldi procedure [25] or its modern modification [26] involves percutaneous drainage of the bulla using a balloon catheter to prevent migration of the drainage tube following prior talc pleurodesis to ensure that the bulla is adherent to the chest wall and does fall away on deflation, leading to pneumothorax. In my experience, this procedure does run the risk of a persistent air leak. That is why I would favour the additional insertion of endobronchial valves. But most patients will tolerate minimally invasive bullectomy using spontaneous ventilation if possible.

8.3 Lung Cancer and Emphysema

We have talked about the complications of emphysematous bullae, but one must not forget the potential for associated malignant change.

Of course. The two conditions share the same aetiological agent, and in lung cancer screening, an abnormality in the wall of a bulla must not be dismissed as inflammatory. Similarly, the resected bullectomy specimen must be subjected to histological analysis, even in younger patients, since occult lung cancer may be detected [27].

As you say, lung cancer and emphysema are frequently associated, so have any of the lessons learned from LVR affected lung cancer surgery?

Yes. The major co-morbidity in smokers under assessment for lung cancer surgery is COPD and severe emphysema is likely to be the most common reason for inoperability due to concerns about the patients' ability to tolerate further lung resection. However, there still seems to be a lack of appreciation for the benefits of LVR. As an example, the latest guidelines for fitness for lung cancer treatment make no mention of LVR [28].

I suppose that is because LVR is not widely practised and respiratory physicians who specialize in COPD are not necessarily involved in lung cancer management. But how would you integrate the knowledge from LVR into lung cancer surgery?

Firstly, in the assessment of patients with lung cancer for resection, the predicted postoperative lung function was based on segment counting of the required resection [29]. This assumption of equal distribution of function, particularly in those with emphysema, is now invalidated. The appreciation of interlobar and intralobar heterogeneity of disease and function, as shown in perfusion scans [30] are now understood.

So, patients with lung cancer and emphysema may be able to lose more lung tissue than previously thought without such a detrimental effect on postoperative lung function. But LVRS does not normally involve anatomical lung resection, so are the two types of surgery compatible?

Certainly. There are three main operative strategies to apply the benefits of LVR to lung cancer surgery. Lobar resection of an emphysematous lobe containing the tumour has been shown to be safe and leaves the patient without severe limitation due to the benefit of improved pulmonary mechanics [31]. If lobectomy is not feasible, then sublobar resection as part of the peripheral "shaving" in conventional LVRS is possible and therapeutic so long as tumour resection margins are respected [32]. Finally, the LVR procedure can be directed at the non-lung cancer target part of the lung to improve lung function to allow the conventional lung cancer resection elsewhere. The LVR functional improvement offsets the loss of functioning tissue due to the cancer. The concomitant LVR can be surgical or endobronchial [33, 34].

But the risk of postoperative complications must be increased by operating on these patients with severe COPD?

Of course, prolonged air leak (PAL), defined as an air leak that persists beyond postoperative day 5, is consistently associated with COPD. Similarly, COPD is a risk factor for postoperative pneumonia [35]. However, as we have discussed in Chapter 7, the risks of LVRS have been overestimated, but it is not unreasonable to use these outcomes when consenting and preparing a patient with severe emphysema for lung cancer surgery, provided a similar work-up has been completed. Lung cancer resection rates increase when the unit also offers LVRS [36, 37].

8.4 Conclusions

Even if one does not practice LVR routinely, then the application of its underlying principles can have a positive effect on more common conditions. In cases of SSP, the surgeon may be more encouraged to operate if the patient is hyperinflated and the air leak arises from an emphysematous lobe. Similarly, the presence of a "giant" bulla may not instill such fear of the lung never fully re-expanding after bullectomy. An understanding of the underlying pathophysiology may present the opportunity to significantly improve the patient's quality of life.

In lung cancer surgery I believe that the most important contributory factor to the increase in the resection rate in the UK has been the appreciation that standard predictors of postoperative lung function may have been unnecessarily pessimistic. The understanding is that if the tumour lies within an emphysematous area of lung, there may be the opportunity to resect it without significant detrimental effects.

References

1 Hallifax RJ, Goldacre R, Landray MJ, Rahman NM, Goldacre MJ. Trends in the incidence and recurrence of inpatient-treated spontaneous pneumothorax, 1968–2016. JAMA. 2018 Oct 9;320(14):1471–1480.
2 Bobbio A, Dechartres A, Bouam S, Damotte D, Rabbat A, Régnard J-F, et al. Epidemiology of spontaneous pneumothorax: gender-related differences. Thorax. 2015;70(7):653–658.
3 Chee CB, Abisheganaden J, Yeo JK, Lee P, Huan PY, Poh SC, et al. Persistent air-leak in spontaneous pneumothorax--clinical course and outcome. Respir Med. 1998 May;92(5):757–761.
4 Onuki T, Ueda S, Yamaoka M, Sekiya Y, Yamada H, Kawakami N, et al. Primary and secondary spontaneous pneumothorax: prevalence, clinical features, and in-hospital mortality. Can Respir. J. 2017; 2017:6014967.
5 Walker SP, Keenan E, Bintcliffe O, Stanton AE, Roberts M, Pepperell J, et al. Ambulatory management of secondary spontaneous pneumothorax: a randomised controlled trial. Eur Respir J. 2021;57(6):2003375.
6 Walker S, Hallifax R, Ricciardi S, Fitzgerald D, Keijzers M, Lauk O, et al. Joint ERS/EACTS/ESTS clinical practice guidelines on adults with spontaneous pneumothorax. Eur J Cardiothorac Surg. 2024;65(5):ezae189.
7 Mathur R, Cullen J, Kinnear WJ, Johnston ID. Time course of resolution of persistent air leak in spontaneous pneumothorax. Respir Med. 1995;89(2): 129–132.
8 Videm V, Pillgram-Larsen J, Ellingsen O, Andersen G, Ovrum E. Spontaneous pneumothorax in chronic obstructive pulmonary disease: complications, treatment and recurrences. Eur J Respir Dis. 1987;71(5):365–371.
9 Baumann MH, Strange C, Heffner JE, Light R, Kirby TJ, Klein J, et al. Management of spontaneous pneumothorax: an American College of Chest Physicians Delphi consensus statement. Chest. 2001;119(2):590–602.
10 Waller DA, McConnell SA, Rajesh PB. Delayed referral reduces the success of video-assisted thoracoscopic surgery for spontaneous pneumothorax. Respir Med. 1998;92(2):246–249.
11 Waller DA, Forty J, Soni AK, Conacher ID, Morritt GN. Videothoracoscopic operation for secondary spontaneous pneumothorax. Ann Thorac Surg. 1994; 57(6):1612–1615.

12 Ibrahim IM, Elaziz MEA, El-Hag-Aly MA. Early autologous blood-patch pleurodesis versus conservative management for treatment of secondary spontaneous pneumothorax. Thorac Cardiovasc Surg. 2019;67(3):222–226.

13 Cao Gq, Kang J, Wang F, Wang H. Intrapleural instillation of autologous blood for persistent air leak in spontaneous pneumothorax in patients with advanced chronic obstructive pulmonary disease. Ann Thorac Surg. 2012;93(5):1652–1657.

14 Fiorelli A, D'Andrilli A, Cascone R, Occhiati L, Anile M, Diso D, et al. Unidirectional endobronchial valves for management of persistent air-leaks: results of a multicenter study. J Thorac Dis. 2018;10(11):61586167.

15 Smesseim I, Morin-Thibault LV, Herth FJF, Tonkin J, Shah PL, Slebos DJ, et al. Endobronchial valves in treatment of persistent air leak: European case-series study and best practice recommendations – from an expert panel. Respiration. 2024;103(9):544–562.

16 Hou G, Wang W, Wang QY, Kang J. Bronchoscopic bullectomy with a one-way endobronchial valve to treat a giant bulla in an emphysematous lung: a case report. Clin Respir J. 2016 Sep;10(5):657–660.

17 Lee EG, Rhee CK. Bronchoscopic lung volume reduction using an endobronchial valve to treat a huge emphysematous bulla: a case report. BMC Pulm Med. 2019 May 14;19(1):92.

18 Santini M, Fiorelli A, Vicidomini G, Di Crescenzo VG, Messina G, Laperuta P. Endobronchial treatment of giant emphysematous bullae with one-way valves: a new approach for surgically unfit patients. Eur J Cardiothorac Surg. 2011;40(6):1425–1431.

19 Tian Q, An Y, Xiao BB, Chen LA. Treatment of giant emphysematous bulla with endobronchial valves in patients with chronic obstructive pulmonary disease: a case series. J Thorac Dis. 2014;6(12):1674–1680.

20 Ballay N, Soder B, Smith J, Miller A, Headrick JR Jr. Intrabronchial pneumonectomy for vanishing lung syndrome: first reported case. Ann Thorac Surg. 2017;103(3):e27 7–e279.

21 Goud A, Krimsky W, Caldwell M, et al. Percutaneous bullectomy in conjunction with endobronchial valve placement as an alternative to surgical management of giant bullae. Respiration. 2016;91(6):523–526.

22 Zoumot Z, Kemp SV, Caneja C, Singh S, Shah PL. Bronchoscopic intrabullous autologous blood instillation: a novel approach for the treatment of giant bullae. Ann Thorac Surg. 2013;96(4):1488–1491.

23 Lee KH, Cho SJ, Ryu SM, Park SM, Yie KS, Han SS. Fluid-filled giant bulla treated with percutaneous drainage and talc sclerotherapy: a modified Brompton technique. Korean J Thorac Cardiovasc Surg. 2012;45(2):134–137.

24 Takanami I. Endoscopic drainage of an infected giant bulla. Interact Cardiovasc Thorac Surg. 2006;5(6):794–795.

25 Head JR, Avery EE. Intracavitary suction (Monaldi) in the treatment of emphysematous bullae and blebs. J Thorac Surg. 1949 Dec;18(6):761–776, illust; Disc, 798–803.

26 Shah SS, Goldstraw P. Surgical treatment of bullous emphysema: experience with the Brompton technique. Ann Thorac Surg. 1994;58(5):1452–1456.

27 Lee M, Dhanji AR, Santhirakumaran G, Perikleous P, Waller D. Incidental finding of lung adenocarcinoma following routine bullectomy and pleurodesis on a young patient: a case report. JRSM Open. 2025;16(5):20542704241304218.

28 Brunelli A, Hardavella G, Huber RM, Berghmans T, Frille A, Rodriguez M, et al. European respiratory society and European society of thoracic surgeons clinical practice guideline on fitness for curative intent treatment of lung cancer. Eur Respir J. 2025;66(5):2500156.

29 Zeiher BG, Gross TJ, Kern JA, Lanza LA, Peterson MW. Predicting postoperative pulmonary function in patients undergoing lung resection. Chest. 1995;108(1):68–72.

30 Ju JW, Suh M, Choi H, Na KJ, Park S, Cheon GJ, et al. Clinical factors affecting discrepancy between predicted and long-term actual lung function following surgery. Clin Nucl Med. 2024;49(11):e574–e579.

31 Edwards JG, Duthie DJ, Waller DA. Lobar volume reduction surgery: a method of increasing the lung cancer resection rate in patients with emphysema. Thorax. 2001;56(10):791–795.

32 Choong CK, Mahesh B, Patterson GA, Cooper JD. Concomitant lung cancer resection and lung volume reduction surgery. Thorac Surg Clin. 2009;19(2):209–216.

33 Fiorelli A, Leonardi B, Messina G, Luzzi L, Paladini P, Catelli C, et al. Lung resection for non-small cell lung cancer following bronchoscopic lung volume reduction for heterogenous emphysema. Cancers (Basel). 2024;16(3):605.

34 Perikleous P, Bilancia R, Oey I, Waller DA. Hybrid bilobectomy for treatment of an early-stage lung cancer in a patient with severe emphysema using the benefits of lung volume reduction. Eur J Cardiothorac Surg. 2017;52(5):1000–1002.

35 Ahuja J, Agrawal R, Strange CD, Price MC, Shroff GS, Truong MT, et al. Postoperative complications in lung cancer. Radiol Clin North Am. 2025;63(4):565–581.

36 Martin-Ucar AE, Waller DA, Atkins JL, Swinson D, O'Byrne KJ, Peake MD. The beneficial effects of specialist thoracic surgery on the resection rate for non-small-cell lung cancer. Lung Cancer. 2004;46(2):227–232.

37 Lau KK, Rathinam S, Waller DA, Peake MD. The effects of increased provision of thoracic surgical specialists on the variation in lung cancer resection rate in England. J Thorac Oncol. 2013;8(1):68–72.

9

From Remodelling to Replacement

9.1 Relative Benefits

LVR surgeon: Chronic obstructive pulmonary disease (COPD), including alpha-1 antitrypsin deficiency, constitutes one of the most common indications for lung transplant worldwide [1]. Do you see lung volume reduction and lung transplantation to be complementary interventions for COPD or are they both options for some patients?

Transplant surgeon: Evidence shows that both procedures can significantly improve lung function, quality of life and survival when patients are carefully selected. Despite some overlap in indication criteria, most patients qualify for only one of the procedures, based on their specific clinical constellation.

Are there any direct comparisons of LVR and LTx?

There is no direct comparative data in similar patient cohorts, but in a meta-analysis of over 3,500 patients in 65 prospective series (where age was not significantly different at 60 years), LTx resulted in a greater perioperative improvement in FEV_1, and overall survival was similar [2].

That's very interesting. So, what is the indication for LTx in emphysema then?

Well, don't forget that the disease severity, as evidenced by worse airflow obstruction, is far worse in those undergoing LTx. at selection. So, there is increased early mortality, and the overall cost of LTx is higher than LVRS, reflecting longer hospital stay and more complicated follow-up. [3].

Yes, that makes sense, but more experienced LVR services are pushing the boundaries of selection into traditional contraindications such as pulmonary hypertension or homogeneous emphysema.

9.2 Selection Criteria

Are there not some factors which would almost certainly preclude LVR and mandate transplant referral?

Certainly, severe hypercapnia with pCO_2 7.5–8 kPa and hypoxia with $pO_2 < 6$ kPa.

What about the BODE index?

LVR may be considered for a BODE index of 7, but probably only in an elderly patient of over 60 years. We found that LVRS in the over 60s in the higher risk categories was surprisingly beneficial. In a series of patients undergoing LVRS, we compared the outcomes of 109 patients (54 male: 55 female) with a BODE index of 6 or less with 47 patients (34 male: 13 female) with a BODE of 7–9 (Figures 9.1–9.3). [4]. Those in the higher BODE index group, who would otherwise have been LTx candidates, had significant improvements in physiology and quality of life. A similar finding was demonstrated when the patients were categorized by the

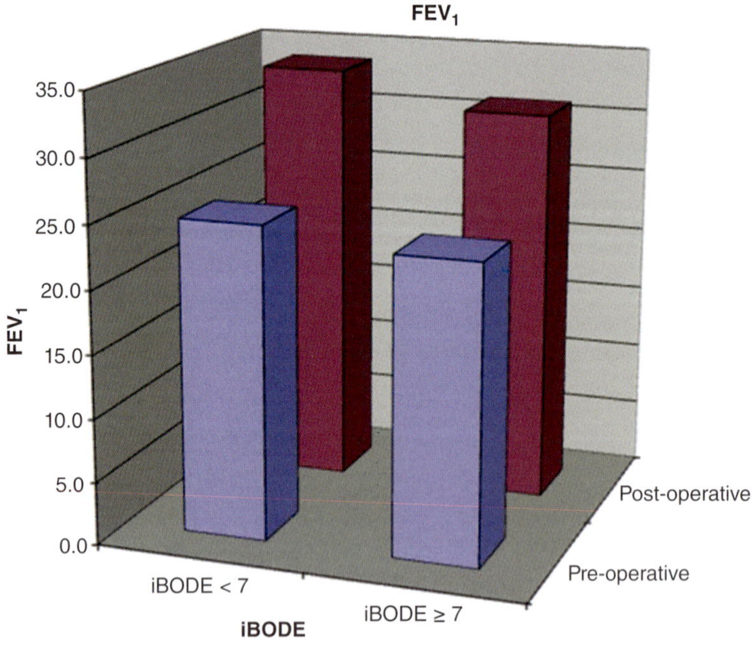

Figure 9.1 The perioperative change in FEV_1 after LVRS in groups with a BODE index above and below 7.

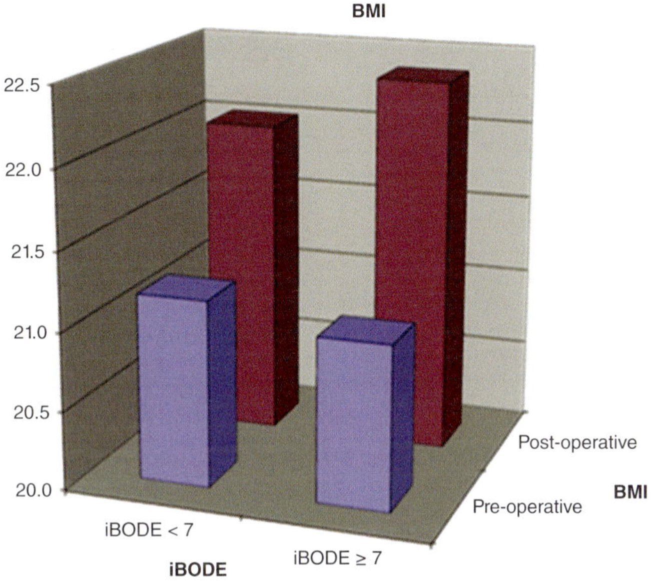

Figure 9.2 The perioperative change in body mass index (BMI) after LVRS in groups with BODE index above and below 7.

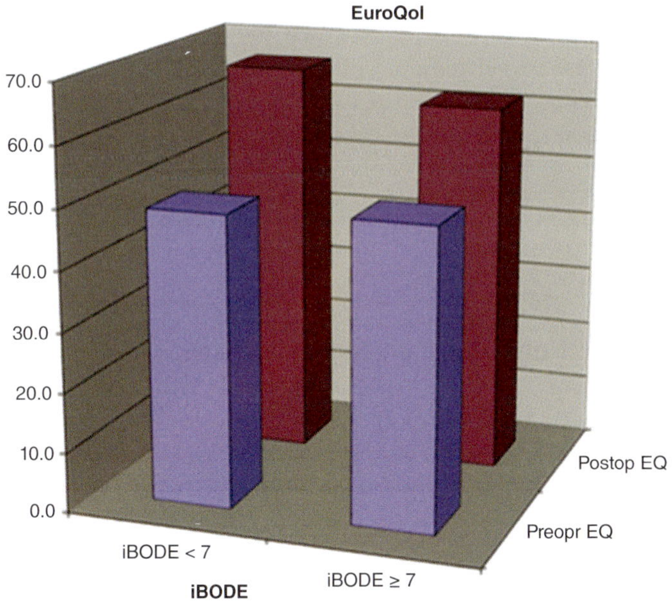

Figure 9.3 The perioperative change in EuroQol after LVRS in groups with BODE index above and below 7.

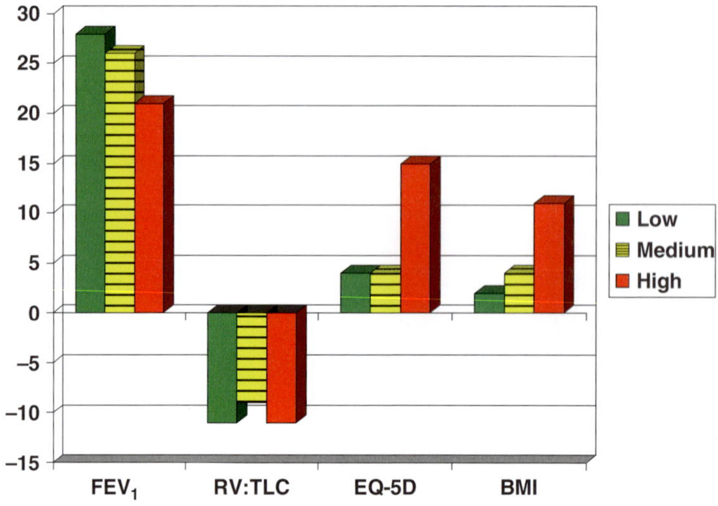

Figure 9.4 The perioperative changes in physiology and quality of life after LVRS in groups with increasing risk scores.

Glenfield BFG risk score [5], where those at most risk had the most gain (Figure 9.4).

In a younger patient, that severity should prompt a transplant referral [6]. However, this decision may depend on the likelihood of the patient obtaining a donor organ in that specific healthcare setting.

We would support the preferential treatment with LVR in those patients over 65 years or those with impaired renal function or mild to moderate coronary artery disease.

9.3 Combining LVR and Lung Transplantation

In the setting of reduced availability of donor organs, how do you feel about the use of LVRS or EBLVR as a temporizing measure as a "bridge" to transplantation?

I am a little concerned that it may compromise the conduct of the subsequent transplant. Previous LVRS can lead to pleural adhesions and may complicate the recipient pneumonectomy with increased risk of bleeding and prolonged operating and therefore ischaemic times [7].

I think that the use of minimally invasive surgery for LVRS and modifications in the materials for buttressing the staple lines may significantly reduce the problem of pleural adhesions. And of course, more patients are receiving EBLVR now.

There is less experience with LTx after EBLVR, but there is a suggestion of a higher incidence of bacterial colonization of the airways compared to non-LVR controls and possibly more postoperative wound infections [8].

But in those borderline patients, at the better end of the spectrum, LVR can postpone the need for LTx, and by improving their functional and nutritional status, can optimize them for future transplant surgery. However, for younger patients, a single LTx procedure may offer immediately greater functional improvement with similar long-term survival [9].

Agreed. In fact, LVRS does not technically compromise the possibility of LTx nor does it impair post-LTx survival in patients with severe COPD. So LVRS for LTx should always be considered for highly selected patients in whom they would not only have a quality of life and functional benefit from LVRS but possibly a reduced peri-operative risk after future LTx.

And of course, if LVRS can delay the need for transplantation, then that is a significant advantage given the shortage of donor organs.

That is a problem for patients with COPD as they may not be of the highest priority when it comes to the allocation of donor lungs [10]. Furthermore, it was found that nearly 5% died while waiting, and another 5% were removed due to clinical deterioration [11].

On that subject, somewhat controversially, how do you feel about combining the benefits of LVR and transplantation and reverting to a single lung transplant (SLTx) for COPD?

Certainly, unrestricted listing for possible single or double LTx may reduce the mortality whilst waiting, particularly in those with significant pulmonary hypertension. But posttransplant survival is better after DLTx (median survival, 6.5 vs 5.3 years and 10-year survival, 33.8% vs 21.6%) [11]. This has been borne out in a more recent meta-analysis [12]. However, survival needs to be measured from the date of listing, not just after the transplant operation.

So, is it better to wait for a DLTx or go for an SLTx sooner if you have severe emphysema?

For the older recipient, it is probably better to accept a single LTx, but we are concerned about complications from the contralateral native emphysematous lung.

What are the main concerns?

In the immediate postoperative period, particularly when the patient is subject to mechanical ventilation, there is a problem with the differential compliance of the two lungs. Preferential expansion of the native lung can lead to mediastinal shift and haemodynamic instability. There is also a real risk of a ventilation/perfusion mismatch. The transplanted organ has better perfusion, but the native lung receives most of the tidal volume.

I guess this is where early or even concurrent lung volume reduction could help?

Possibly, but there are also the later potential problems with infection in the native side from either intrinsic pneumonia or extrinsic from prolonged air leak and drainage. There is also a more delayed risk of malignancy in the native lung due to the smoking history and future immunosuppression. These late native lung complications contribute to the comparatively better survival from a double lung transplant.

So, can we help by performing LVR on the native lung after SLTx?

It may have a role as both LVRS and EBLVR have been used after single LTx to improve overall lung function and reduce native lung complications. A pneumothorax and persistent air leak have been treated with endobronchial valves [13]. Compensatory hyperinflation of the native lung has been successfully treated by endobronchial methods [14] and by LVRS [15] or lobectomy [16]. But there are always concerns regarding infective complications from prolonged drainage after native lung operations in immunosuppressed patients.

In conclusion, I assume that you would advocate the involvement of the lung transplant team in the lung volume reduction network?

Ideally, yes, but the relative scarcity of lung transplant programmes may make the proposal of incorporating a transplant surgeon into each LVR MDT unworkable. However, each MDT should have an identified lung transplant programme associated with it and a robust method of intercommunication.

So, what advice would you have for the LVR MDT?

I think that lung transplantation is intended to treat end-stage emphysema patients where all other interventions fail, so that LVR techniques should be explored wherever possible, including in the higher-risk groups. However, there is no problem in referring these borderline patients for transplant assessment in the interim. Of course, those in whom LVR is contraindicated with frequent infective exacerbations or who have developed respiratory failure should be diverted from the LVR MDT to the nearest transplant centre.

I think the message is that LVR and lung transplant are complementary rather than competing options, and closer links are important between the respective teams are to be encouraged.

I think we should illustrate the complementary, symbiotic relationship between the LVR MDT and the lung transplant team with three clinical cases.

9.4 Illustrative Case Studies

9.4.1 Case 1 – Young Patient, Very Bad Emphysema

This 45-year-old male smoked cannabis heavily for 20 years until his late thirties, but has no other comorbidities. He has no other history of drug abuse and has negative viral serology.

He is extremely breathless with an MRC score of 5. He is significantly hyperinflated with his RV 340% predicted.

That sounds like the ideal LVR candidate.

Not so fast. His BODE index is 7 as he has lost weight, and his FEV_1 is only 19% predicted.

So still LVR material, if a little high risk.

His very big lungs are severely emphysematous with upper and lower lobe disease and little heterogeneity.

But I thought that you could still benefit from LVR even in so-called homogeneous emphysema if there was such extreme hyperinflation?

True, but he is becoming hypercapnic with his pCO_2 hovering over 7 kPa and his pO_2 is only a little higher at 7.2 kPa.

I thought that successful LVR could reduce hypercapnia? What about his cardiac function?

OK, his hypercapnia is a relative contraindication, but his right heart is failing with right ventricular dilatation and moderate pulmonary hypertension on transthoracic echocardiography.

Sounds less and less suitable for LVR.

I suppose that we could probably offer unilateral LVRS to bridge him to a future lung transplant.

No, I think straight to lung transplant assessment as the odds are stacking up against him. However, in those who survive for over 1 year, transplant has a higher level of functional status, greater improvement in airflow obstruction, dyspnoea, exercise tolerance, and BODE index. I would be concerned that likely complications from LVR may risk his chance of a successful transplant.

9.4.2 Case 2 – Moderate Risk, Just Bad Enough?

This 55-year-old male, who stopped cigarette smoking five years ago, has recently lost his job after two AECOPD episodes in the last 12 months. He has an MRC score of 4 and a BODE index of 5–6.

How suitable is he for LVR?

He is very hyperinflated; RV 270% predicted and has bilateral upper lobe target areas. But he is heading towards frequent exacerbations.

So why not go for LVR?

He is of moderate to high risk with FEV_1 20% predicted and DLCO 21% predicted.

Is he in respiratory failure?

Well, his pO2 is 9 kPa, but his pCO_2 is 6.8 kPa.

So maybe too good for transplant at present. What can you tell me about his cardiac function?

His estimated mean pulmonary artery pressure is 35 mmHg, but there is no suggestion of right ventricular dysfunction.

Sounds like a possible transplant candidate, but would you consider LVR?

Yes, but should we intend it as a bridge and concurrently work up for both LVR and transplant?

I agree.

9.4.3 Case 3 – Too Bad for Any Treatment?

The final case is one of a 65-year-old female, an ex-smoker again, who is hyperinflated with her RV 240% predicted. She is severely breathless with MRC 4–5 and BODE 6.

So still suitable for LVR.

Yes, but high risk with FEV_1 20% predicted and DLCO 24% predicted.

How about her blood gas analysis?

She has required nocturnal non-invasive ventilation, but her pCO_2 at present is 6.6 KPa and her pO_2 8.2 KPa.

Does she have any cardiac problems?

On transthoracic echocardiography, she has borderline pulmonary hypertension with mild right ventricular dysfunction. Also, with a chronic history of hypertension, her left ventricular ejection fraction is mildly reduced.

Does she have any renal impairment?

Yes, attributed to the hypertension. Her serum creatinine is mildly elevated, and her glomerular filtration rate is mildly reduced.

I think the balance is tipping away from transplantation due to her age and comorbidity, which will increase the risk of transplantation and cause subsequent problems with immunosuppression. I am particularly concerned about her borderline renal impairment and possible coronary artery disease with left ventricular dysfunction [17].

Does she have targets for LVR?

Yes, clear upper lobe predominant disease and a 100% intact left major interlobar fissure. So, on balance, I favour Left EBLVR as the definitive treatment.

Agreed, there is no benefit from waiting for an organ to become available whilst using the EBLVR as a bridge. She may be almost 70 years old when this becomes possible, and her renal function may have deteriorated further.

9.5 Conclusions

Lung transplantation offers the hope of extended survival to patients in the end-stage of chronic lung disease. However, COPD is only one of many indications for this treatment. The overlap with LVR and transplantation relates to a typically middle-aged population that has reached end-staged emphysema after smoking cigarettes for most of their adult life. The relative benefits of transplantation in this cohort are likely to be less than in the younger population with end-stage fibrotic, infective or pulmonary vascular disease. So, in a situation of donor lung limitation, it is not unreasonable to ask is there not an alternative for the emphysema patients, thus releasing more organs for other indications.

As there appears to be evidence that prior LVR does not prejudice the outcome of a subsequent transplant would not initial remodelling of the damaged organ be the logical first step. However, by definition, these LVR procedures are in those at the worse end of the spectrum. It would seem ideal if these patients were assessed and treated by teams who also can offer lung transplantation. Benefits in joint case assessment and perioperative care would follow.

References

1 Chambers DC, Cherikh WS, Goldfarb SB, Hayes D Jr, Kucheryavaya AY, Toll AE, Khush et al. The International Thoracic Organ Transplant Registry of the International Society for Heart and Lung Transplantation: thirty-fifth adult lung and heart-lung transplant report-2018; focus theme: multiorgan transplantation. J Heart Lung Transplant. 2018;37(10):1169–1183.

2 Ahmad D, Ferrell BE, Saxena A, Jimenez DC, O'Malley TJ, Dispagna MA, et al. Comparative outcomes of lung volume reduction surgery and lung transplantation: a systematic review and meta-analysis. J Thorac Dis. 2023;15(7):3627–3635.

3 Weinstein MS, Martin UJ, Crookshank AD, Chatila W, Vance GB, Gaughan JP, et al. Mortality and functional performance in severe emphysema after lung volume reduction or transplant. COPD. 2007;4(1):15–22.

4 Greening NJ, Vaughan P, Oey I, Steiner MC, Morgan MD, Rathinam S, et al. Individualised risk in patients undergoing lung volume reduction surgery: the Glenfield BFG score. Eur Respir J. 2017;49(6):1601766.

5 Tenconi S, Oey I, Abdulmajid U, Rathinam S, Waller D. Lung volume reduction surgery in lung transplant candidates. Is it worthwhile? Interactive CardioVascular and Thoracic Surgery 2014; 18(S1):S16.

6 Leard LE, Holm AM, Valapour M, Glanville AR, Attawar S, Aversa M, et al. Consensus document for the selection of lung transplant candidates: an update from the International Society for Heart and Lung Transplantation. J Heart Lung Transplant. 2021;40(11):1349–1379.

7 Slama A, Ceulemans LJ, Hedderich C, Boehm PM, Van Slambrouck J, Schwarz S, et al. Lung volume reduction followed by lung transplantation in emphysema: a multicenter matched analysis. Transpl Int. 2022;35:10048.

8 Slama A, Taube C, Kamler M, Aigner C. Lung volume reduction followed by lung transplantation-considerations on selection criteria and outcome. J Thorac Dis. 2018 Oct;10(Suppl 27):S3366–S3375. https://doi.org/10.21037/jtd.2018.06.164

9 Inci I, Iskender I, Ehrsam J, Caviezel C, Hillinger S, Opitz I, et al. Previous lung volume reduction surgery does not negatively affect survival after lung transplantation. Eur J Cardiothorac Surg. 2018 Mar 1;53(3): 596–602. https://doi.org/10.1093/ejcts/ezx318

10 Egan TM, Edwards LB. Effect of the lung allocation score on lung transplantation in the United States. J Heart Lung Transplant. 2016;35(4):433–439.
11 Hull TD, Leya GA, Axtell AL, Moonsamy P, Osho A, Chang DC, et al. Lung transplantation for chronic obstructive pulmonary disease: a call to modify the lung allocation score to decrease waitlist mortality. J Thorac Cardiovasc Surg. 2022;164(4):1222–1233.e11.
12 Fang YC, Cheng WH, Lu HI, Wang YS, Chuang KH, Lai HH, et al. Double lung transplantation is better than single lung transplantation for end-stage chronic obstructive pulmonary disease: a meta-analysis. J Cardiothorac Surg. 2024;19(1):162.
13 Godts J, Etienne I, Knoop C, Leduc D, Sokolow Y, Vander Kuylen M, et al. Endobronchial valve treatment for persistent air leak and endoscopic lung volume reduction of native lung in a single lung transplant recipient: a case report and literature review. Respirol Case Rep. 2025;13(8):e70305. https://doi.org/10.1002/rcr2.70305
14 Perch M, Jensen K, Kalhauge A, Hansen HJ, Mortensen J. A case of native lung hyperinflation after single lung transplantation treated with lung volume reduction coils. JHLT Open. 2024;5:100103. https://doi.org/10.1016/j.jhlto.2024.100103
15 Wilson H, Carby M, Beddow E. Lung volume reduction surgery for native lung hyperinflation following single-lung transplantation for emphysema: which patients? Eur J Cardiothorac Surg. 2012;42(3):410–413. https://doi.org/10.1093/ejcts/ezs086
16 Reece TB, Mitchell JD, Zamora MR, Fullerton DA, Cleveland JC, Pomerantz M, et al. Native lung volume reduction surgery relieves functional graft compression after single-lung transplantation for chronic obstructive pulmonary disease. J Thorac Cardiovasc Surg. 2008 Apr;135(4):931–937. https://doi.org/10.1016/j.jtcvs.2007.10.069
17 Verleden GM, Gottlieb J. Lung transplantation for COPD/pulmonary emphysema. Eur Respir Rev. 2023;32(167):220116. https://doi.org/10.1183/16000617.0116-2022

10

Conclusions

10.1 Increasing the Lung Volume Reduction Referral Base

Administrator: Why is it that we don't see many patients undergoing lung volume reduction (LVR) when COPD is such a common reason for hospital admission?

LVR surgeon: That is a very good question and one which we have posed for nearly 30 years.

Is it a problem of supply or demand?

The demand is undoubtedly out there, and we can discuss issues of supply, in terms of organization of services, later. But the key issue is the pathway by which the large number of patients suitable for LVR reach the teams offering the service.

How large is the potential demand for LVR?

In a study from Boston [1], 15% of patients in a pulmonary function test laboratory database with stages III and IV Global Initiative for Chronic Obstructive Lung Disease (GOLD) had lung volumes, carbon monoxide diffusing capacity and CT scans favourable for LVRS.

That's potentially an enormous number of people. Why is it that LVR options are not considered as part of the standard assessment for COPD?

Well, the latest Global Initiative for Obstructive Lung Disease (GOLD) report [2] recommends LVR as an alternative when inhaled therapies and pulmonary rehabilitation have already been used to maximal effect,

so most respiratory specialists should be aware of the possibility. This is an internationally recognized report from a group affiliated to the World Health Organization, so it is widely disseminated and respected.

So, are they fearful of LVR?

I believe that some respiratory specialists may be scared. An inappropriate over-estimation of the risks leads to a sense of nihilism towards LVR as a treatment. Hence, the most breathless COPD patients are prematurely discharged from secondary care. They are then managed solely in primary care settings where, for obvious reasons, specialist knowledge of LVR may be lacking [3]. It has been noted that even following the completion and promotion of the National Emphysema Treatment Trial (NETT) findings in the United States and despite the potential life-changing benefits of LVRS, only a low number of procedures are actually performed [4]. So this problem spans different healthcare systems.

How would you address this problem and get more patients through to the LVR services?

I think we can consider four target areas: primary care practices, pulmonary rehabilitation classes, secondary care beds and the, as yet unknown, number who attend lung cancer screening units.

10.1.1 Primary Care

Many patients with COPD are managed in nurse-led clinics [5], having reached the maximal level of pharmacological therapy. This is clearly a target population, and therefore, nursing practitioners must be fully informed of the possibilities associated with LVR. They also need clear referral pathways into secondary care.

A review of a typical rural primary care practice identified that around 3% of those registered with COPD were potentially suitable for LVR [6]. These patients were more socioeconomically deprived and had a higher annual primary care health usage of nearly 50 visits per year. Therefore, they are well known to their primary care physician.

But this population would need more careful selection before being considered for LVR.

Yes, but even if only a small proportion were eventually selected for LVR, this would still be a huge potential surgical workload.

10.1.2 Pulmonary Rehabilitation

These community-based, physiotherapy-led pulmonary rehabilitation (PR) programmes are another potential source of patients with LVR. An audit of the UK COPD practice estimated that of around 15,000 patients, between 5% and 18% may be suitable for further LVR assessment on the basis of their walking distance, baseline spirometry and Medical Research Council (MRC) dyspnoea score [7]. Not all were likely to be sufficiently hyperinflated but those who were would fulfil most of the preliminary requirements.

So these patients who would already be further on in the selection pathway for LVR are particularly symptomatic, have achieved the minimum exercise tolerance?

Yes, this would undoubtedly be the ideal starting point. However, the availability of PR programs is limited, and many LVR-suitable patients may get to the stage of LVR referral before attending such a programme.

10.1.3 Non-elective Admission With an Acute Exacerbation of COPD

Acute exacerbation of COPD (AECOPD) is the second most common cause of emergency admission to hospital and is one of the costliest diseases in terms of acute hospital care in England. In the year 2023–2024 in the United Kingdom, there were over 120,000 hospital admissions with AECOPD, an increase of 9% on the previous year [8].

And how many of these would be suitable for LVR?

I am not aware of any figures, but in our experience, the initial entry onto the LVR pathway for the vast majority came after their first admission with an exacerbation. These patients will have had imaging so hyperinflation can be detected, and they are known to secondary care services. Those in severe cardiac or respiratory failure can be excluded, but the remainder can begin assessment.

That sounds like an ideal plan, so why aren't more referred this way?

The admission is usually transient, and only around one in four patients with AECOPD are admitted to a respiratory ward, so the majority may get no specialist intervention or follow-up. Thirty percent of services report no specialty triage of acute admissions to respiratory medicine. Between 27% and 46% of services report no access to early or supported discharge for acutely

admitted patients (outreach or inreach models, respectively) [9]. They will be given "rescue packs" of an antibiotic and steroid tablets to manage further exacerbations and be followed up largely in primary care.

So, what would you suggest?

I think that there should be a method of alerting the local respiratory services by an electronic system for every admission of AECOPD into their hospital. It may be impossible for every patient to be reviewed by a specialist doctor, but trained nurse practitioners could triage those who may benefit from further specialist follow-up, including those hyperinflated for LVR.

10.1.4 Lung Cancer Screening

The Targeted Lung Health Check (TLHC) with low-dose CT scan was recommended in the United Kingdom by the National Screening Committee in 2022 for patients between the ages of 55 and 74 who are ever smokers. The screening has had the main aim of detecting lung cancer at an early stage; however, several other conditions have been incidentally diagnosed.

I guess that in that population there must be a large percentage of ever smokers with emphysema.

Emphysema is the most common lung incidental finding. During the initial phase, almost 900,000 people were invited for checks, 375,000 risk assessments were made and 200,000 scans were carried out. There were estimated to be around 14,000 with severe emphysema who have got CT scans on the program and thus could be assessed for hyperinflation, heterogeneity and suitability for LVR.

Do they get spirometry at the screening scan?

Not routinely, but of course that would be a good idea.

Are there any international experiences?

Yes, in an American series in a lung cancer screening programme, emphysema was identified by radiologists in two-thirds of cases. Of these, the radiologist graded emphysema severity as mild/minimal 18.6% cases, moderate emphysema in 34.1% cases and severe emphysema in 8.05%. In the total cohort, half of the individuals with emphysema, as determined by radiologist interpretation, had significant airflow obstruction. In fact, there was, of course, a linear correlation exists radiological assessment

of emphysema severity and spirometric values of FEV_1% predicted and DLCO% predicted [10]. In a meta-analysis of 42 studies, the pooled prevalence of emphysema was 45.3%, with moderate to severe emphysema in 28.8%. Significant airflow limitation was found in 40.1% [11].

So, is emphysema screening integrated into the lung cancer screening protocol?

Not really. The addition of screening for cardiovascular disease (coronary artery calcification or aortic enlargement) in a high-risk population offers health benefits at low costs compared with no screening or lung cancer screening alone. But as yet, adding COPD screening cannot be justified owing to the limited clinical evidence, particularly for reduction in mortality [12, 13].

How easy would it be to get a patient from the screening CT into the LVR pathway?

Not as easy as you would hope. Firstly, in most cases (80%), this diagnosis comes as a surprise to patients, who had no previous knowledge of the condition, so it is more likely to cause concern for the patients. Secondly, they need an initial assessment for medical therapy, lifestyle advice and education. There is a discussion about who should bear the brunt of this extra workload, either primary or secondary care. Before any increase in referral for LVR is seen in the tertiary centre, there is a potentially massive increase in workload for COPD clinics, lung function laboratories and rehabilitation programmes.

So "harvesting" patients with LVR from the lung screening programmes is like planting an acorn and waiting for the oak tree to grow. In other words, I do not think it will be a quick way of flooding the LVR lists with suitable patients. But it does have long-term promise and will certainly improve the overall management of these patients.

So, where do you think is the best target for increased referral for LVR?

Of these four alternatives, I think that the low-hanging fruit lies in the acute medical wards in that patients are admitted for their first exacerbation. They are undoubtedly breathless and, having had to call for an emergency admission, will also feel bad enough to want something to be done. All that needs to be done is to filter out those with hyperinflation on their imaging. But resident medical doctors need to be aware of the possibility of LVR, and they need to have clearly identified referral pathways to the local respiratory specialists.

Just explain the pathway, then, for potential LVR candidates.

The key is to get these patients discussed at an LVR multidisciplinary team (MDT) meeting. The MDT meeting provides a forum for high-quality case-specific discussion to appraise the risks and benefits to individual patients, to tailor the risk management of the determined route of LVR, either LVRS or endobronchial LVR (EBLVR) [14].

And what information is required to inform this discussion? How much needs to be done by the referring physician?

The referrers need to show that the patient satisfies the basic cardiorespiratory criteria with full lung function tests and echocardiography. Ideally, they should also have an objective assessment of their exercise tolerance with a walk test. These should allow calculation of an individualized risk score or BODE index.

How far should the referrers go towards assessing and excluding patients on the basis of their imaging?

They should perform the initial high resolution CT scan (HRCT) to inform the LVR MDT about target areas and other respiratory diseases. But it should not be the role of the referring clinician to assume inoperability and block the referral. This is an unnecessary triage by those who are inexperienced in the administration of the eventual treatment episode.

10.2 MDT Working

What members constitute the LVR MDT?

The membership of this MDT must include all specialists involved in the assessment and subsequent treatment of the patient, including non-medical input. The core members are: the clinician who will perform the LVR procedure (this may just be the thoracic surgeon but may include the interventional pulmonologist) a COPD specialist physician (who will ensure validity of the workup), a radiologist (who will interpret the imaging including targets and fissure integrity) and the physician who has met with the patient and who can add finer details. Ideally, there should also be allied healthcare professionals, including physiotherapists and nurse specialists, who may have important, specific patient information. It may be advantageous to include an anaesthetist to plan perioperative care requirements, and if available, a member of the local lung transplant team to advise in the borderline LVR cases.

Presumably, the MDT requires administrative assistance?

There must be a robust administrative organization to collate all the referral material from disparate sources, to record the decisions made and to facilitate inter-disciplinary communication often between several different hospitals. The use of a proforma facilitates this process, but it must be kept simple. The last thing a busy referring clinician wants is to be asked to complete what looks like a tax return document simply to get their patient discussed!

I get your point! You have already outlined the role of the referring physician and the information they must make available to the MDT. But what are the MDT to do with this information?

Following the process outlined in Figure 10.1, firstly, they confirm the anatomical and physiological suitability for the procedure and estimate the individual risk. Secondly, they must allocate the appropriate intervention, LVRS or EBLVR, based on imaging of target areas and the likelihood of collateral ventilation. Possible postoperative complications, including the risk of post-EBLVR pneumothorax, can be predicted and a warning flagged. Finally, specific preoperative preparation may need to be made, including optimization of fitness before bronchoscopy or surgery. In more established programmes, there will be a need for rediscussion for second-stage procedures [15].

How often should the MDT meet? What is the optimum use of resources?

The MDT should meet as frequently as possible to keep the momentum of the service moving. Referrers need to see action taken for their patients,

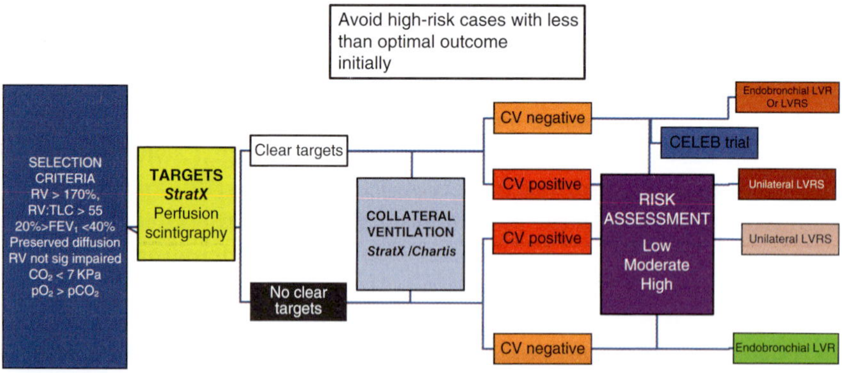

Figure 10.1 A schematic description of the LVR pathway.

and one must avoid large hiatuses in communication. For most practices, a monthly meeting is sufficient.

What about the structure of the MDT?

The meeting should be short and sweet. Probably no more than one hour and around six cases. But for each case, all relevant information should be available. There is nothing more frustrating than cases being put forward for screening purposes with only a few details. This only leads to deferment and repeated discussion at subsequent meetings.

So, is the MDT just a rubber-stamping exercise?

Absolutely not. It has been shown that increased awareness of the referral criteria and pathway has increased the referral numbers for LVR, but also education of referring physicians on selection and outcomes has led to a higher rate of selection of suitable cases. However, the main function of the LVR MDT is to determine the appropriate target for LVR and the most effective method of achieving it.

The MDT will decline referrals then?

Of course, almost all referrals should meet the physiological selection criteria, so the majority of patients are considered unsuitable because of the absence of target areas on a quantitative perfusion scan, which is usually arranged at the treatment (MDT) centre for continuity. The other reason for not progressing to treatment is the appreciation of relative risk. Either the patients were considered too good by the medical team or because the patients felt they were too good to consider LVR at this stage. Less common reasons include: previous thoracic surgery or other associated respiratory conditions, such as frequent exacerbations, bronchiectasis or lung fibrosis [16].

10.3 Organization of LVR Services

OK, so you've created this super-efficient, well-organized LVR MDT. How are you going to get the referrals?

Well, firstly, you have got to get out and "spread the word" with face-to-face promotional meetings at educational events, giving the evidence for LVR in a clear form, illustrated with real-life case studies. There is no future just in sitting in your "ivory tower" and expecting the work to come to you.

Secondly, the service has to be "user-friendly." Keep the selection criteria broad at first. Provide a simple referral proforma and give a single contact referral source managed by a single practitioner to process referrals expeditiously for discussion at the MDT.

Thirdly, give efficient feedback on referrals. Explaining why patients cannot be treated or why a specific method has been chosen results in increased education for the local team and an increase in referrals. Supplement this with regular meetings with referrers, either face-to-face or using remote platforms to widen referral base.

Finally, realize that you are developing a comprehensive service, not just providing one-off technical expertise. There are benefits in establishing a multidisciplinary LVR clinic in the local referral community in conjunction with your referrer. Patient travel is reduced, it makes more use of local investigations, and most importantly, it provides a focal point as patients often feel "cut adrift" once treated.

And how is this working in practice?

Of course, there have been expressions of concern regarding problems with access. This results in a "postcode lottery" as a significant proportion of respiratory physicians reported having limited access to advanced COPD multidisciplinary services and LVR. A survey of members of the British Thoracic Society described an absence of clinical pathways for LVR. Half of the respondents were either unsure about the risks of death, or prolonged (>30 days) hospital stay involved, or significantly overestimated them. 70% did not have a specific multidisciplinary team to discuss the management of patients with advanced COPD [17]. In a patient experience exercise of those who had gone through the LVR process, many described how they "had to fight to get a referral" [18].

So, should LVR be a routine procedure in all thoracic units, not just a niche interest in specialized centres?

That would be the ideal situation, but it is, unfortunately, probably unrealistic. There needs to be a sufficient number of centres to ensure equity of access, but they need to be restricted enough to ensure specialist input. It is true that the need to concentrate LVR procedures and expertise to a limited number of highly specialised means that there is poor geographical coverage throughout countries, contributing to a lack of understanding and consideration for LVR amongst the primary and secondary care communities. This creates a "doom-loop" of reduced knowledge, lower referrals and ultimately fewer interventions being performed. Although in the

United Kingdom, NHS England agreed to widespread commissioning of LVR services, in the United States, certification mandated by the Center for Medicare and Medicaid Services is onerous and expensive, and thus the centres providing LVRS are few and far between [4].

What is your conclusion?

The ideal situation is to have experience concentrated in regional LVR centres, but these have outreach clinics in their referral communities. I have seen the benefits of this model.

10.4 Societal Benefits

This all sounds very impressive, but how am I, as a healthcare administrator, going to justify funding your thoracic surgeons to operate on patients with emphysema?

10.4.1 Return to Work

Aside from the direct cost to the healthcare system from COPD, it is estimated that in the United Kingdom over 24 million working days are lost each year from COPD. This costs an estimated £3.8 billion to the economy through reduced productivity [19]. LVR, by increasing exercise ability, may return those of working age to employment, not only increasing productivity and tax revenue but importantly reducing the cost to society from welfare benefit payments and social care requirements. These patients may not only carrying on working but may also remain in their private residences.

10.4.2 Reduced Hospital Admission

The direct healthcare cost of COPD to the United Kingdom is estimated at over £800 million a year [20]. Acute exacerbations are the cost drivers for COPD care, accounting for more than 70% of COPD-related costs incurred as a result of emergency visits and hospitalisations [21]. LVR reduces admission to the hospital with AECOPD.

In NETT over the first two years of follow-up, patients undergoing LVRS had approximately 33% fewer respiratory hospital admissions per patient-year compared with those managed medically [22]. Similar benefits follow EBLVR of around 30%, particularly if lobar atelectasis is obtained [23].

A very important point to make is that while there is a fourfold variation in non-elective admissions across England, and readmission rates vary by up to five times in different parts of the country [24], UK audit data indicate that centres performing LVRS report sustained reductions in hospital bed-days, driven primarily by fewer emergency admissions for COPD exacerbations in the first 12 months post-surgery compared with the year prior to LVRS [25].

10.4.3 Survival Benefit

But does LVR increase survival or life-expectancy?

Back to the NETT, LVRS resulted in a five-year life expectancy of 63–78%, which was approximately a 10% improvement over medical treatment, and the benefit was higher in the upper-lobe predominant, lower exercise capacity patients [26].

Finally, in the UK Lung Volume Reduction Registry, five-year survival was 75% following LVRS and 71% following EBLVR, which is significantly higher than reported in other severe COPD cohorts that had not undergone an LVR intervention (around 33%). The mean BODE score in this cohort at baseline for those receiving LVRS and EBVs is typically associated with around 57% survival over four years (52 months). In those fulfilling selection criteria, LVR can substantially increase life expectancy [27].

Thank you. You have made a very convincing case for funding the LVR services. Now I would advise the enthusiastic would-be LVR clinicians to take up the challenge.

References

1 Akuthota P, Litmanovich D, Zutler M, Boiselle PM, Bankier AA, Roberts DH, et al. An evidence-based estimate on the size of the potential patient pool for lung volume reduction surgery. Ann Thorac Surg. 2012;94(1):205–211.

2 Global Initiative for Chronic Obstructive Pulmonary Disease. Global strategy for the diagnosis, management and prevention of chronic obstructive pulmonary disease. Annual Report 2026. https://goldcopd.org/2026-gold-report/

3 Mahadeva R, Zoumot Z. Living with COPD: the struggle for breath and for lung volume reduction therapies. ERJ Open Res. 2018;4(2):00005–2018.

4 Naunheim K. Invited commentary. Ann Thorac Surg. 2012;94(1):211.

5 Aranburu-Imatz A, López-Carrasco JC, Moreno-Luque A, Jiménez-Pastor JM, Valverde-León MDR, Rodríguez-Cortés FJ, et al. Nurse-led interventions in chronic obstructive pulmonary disease patients: a systematic review and meta-analysis. Int J Environ Res Public Health. 2022;19(15):9101.

6 Ward TJC, John C, Williams AT, Batini C, Greening NJ, Tobin MD, et al. Identifying eligibility for specialist intervention in COPD from UK primary care data: a "treatable traits" approach. Int J Chron Obstruct Pulmon Dis. 2025; 20:2761–2766.

7 Buttery SC, Lewis A, Kemp SV, Banya W, Quint JK, Steiner MC, et al. Lung volume reduction eligibility in patients with COPD completing pulmonary rehabilitation: results from the UK National Asthma and COPD Audit Programme. BMJ Open. 2020;10(11):e040942.

8 Office for Health Improvement and Disparities. Respiratory Diseases Profile: statistical commentary, June 2025. https://www.gov.uk/government/statistics/update-of-indicators-in-the-respiratory-disease-profile-june-2025

9 Royal College of Physicians. National Respiratory Audit Program. Organisational Audit 2024: COPD data deep dive. June 2024. https://www.rcp.ac.uk/media/tduixkni/nrap_copd_organisation_audit_data_deep_dive_final.pdf

10 Dachert S, Seigo M, Ahearn O, Zhao H, Criner GJ. Emphysema detection by qualitative and quantitative analysis and relationship to spirometric obstruction in an urban comprehensive lung cancer screening programme: the temple healthy chest initiative (THCI) - a retrospective cohort study. BMJ Open. 2025; 15(10):e094268.

11 Choi H, Kwak IY, Oh CR, Goo JM, Yoon SH. Prevalence of airflow limitation and emphysema in lung cancer screening populations: a systematic review and meta-analysis. Chest. 2025;168(1):67–82.

12 Behr CM, Koffijberg H, Degeling K, Vliegenthart R, IJzerman MJ. Can we increase efficiency of CT lung cancer screening by combining with CVD and COPD screening? Results of an early economic evaluation. Eur Radiol. 2022; 32(5):3067–3075.

13 Behr CM, IJzerman MJ, Kip MMA, Groen HJM, Heuvelmans MA, van den Berge M, et al. Model-based cost-utility analysis of combined low-dose computed tomography screening for lung cancer, chronic obstructive pulmonary disease, and cardiovascular disease. JTO Clin Res Rep. 2025;6(5):100813.

14 Oey I, Waller D. The role of the multidisciplinary emphysema team meeting in the provision of lung volume reduction. J Thorac Dis. 2018;10(Suppl 23): S2824–S2829.

15 Chew J, Mahadeva R. The role of a multidisciplinary severe chronic obstructive pulmonary disease hyperinflation service in patient selection for lung volume reduction. J Thorac Dis. 2018 Oct;10(Suppl 27):S3335–S3343.

16 Rathinam S, Oey I, Steiner M, Spyt T, Morgan MD, Waller DA. The role of the emphysema multidisciplinary team in a successful lung volume reduction surgery programme†. Eur J Cardiothorac Surg. 2014 Dec;46(6): 1021–1026; discussion 1026.

17 McNulty W, Jordan S, Hopkinson NS. Attitudes and access to lung volume reduction surgery for COPD – a survey by the British Thoracic Society. BMJ Open Respir Res. 2014;1:e000023.

18 Buttery S, Lewis A, Oey I, Hargrave J, Waller D, Steiner M, et al. Patient experience of lung volume reduction procedures for emphysema: a qualitative service improvement project. ERJ Open Res. 2017 Aug 11;3(3): 00031–2017.

19 Health and Safety Executive. Health and Safety Statistics. Key Figures for Great Britain 2024/25. https://www.hse.gov.uk/statistics/dayslost.htm

20 National Institute for Health and Care Research. Implantable and Wearable Devices for Chronic Obstructive Pulmonary Disease. 3 June 2019. https://www.nihr.ac.uk/implantable-wearable-medical-devices-chronic-obstructive-pulmonary-disease

21 Oostenbrink JB, Rutten-van Mölken MP. Resource use and risk factors in high-cost exacerbations of COPD. Respir Med. 2004 Sep;98(9): 883–891.

22 Washko GR, Fan VS, Ramsey SD, Mohsenifar Z, Martinez F, Make BJ, et al. The effect of lung volume reduction surgery on chronic obstructive pulmonary disease exacerbations. Am J Respir Crit Care Med. 2008 Jan 15;177(2): 164–169.

23 Brock JM, Böhmker F, Schuster PU, Eberhardt R, Gompelmann D, Kontogianni K, et al. Endobronchial lung volume reduction with valves reduces exacerbations in severe emphysema patients. Respir Med. 2023;218:107399.

24 Friebel R, Hauck K, Aylin P, Steventon A. National trends in emergency readmission rates: a longitudinal analysis of administrative data for England between 2006 and 2016. BMJ Open. 2018;8(3):e020325.

25 NHS England Annual Report and Accounts 2023/24. 31 October 2024. https://www.england.nhs.uk/long-read/performance-report-23-24/

26 Criner GJ, Cordova F, Sternberg AL, Martinez FJ. The national emphysema treatment trial (NETT) Part II: lessons learned about lung volume reduction surgery. Am J Respir Crit Care Med. 2011;184(8):881–893.

27 Buttery SC, Lewis A, Alzetani A, Bolton CE, Curtis KJ, Dodd JW, et al. Survival following lung volume reduction procedures: results from the UK Lung Volume Reduction (UKLVR) registry. BMJ Open Respir Res. 2024;11(1):e002092.

Index